Cancer Biomarkers: Ethics, Economics and Society

ANNE BLANCHARD AND ROGER STRAND
(EDITORS)

First published 2017.

Second printing 2018.

Megaloceros Press is a publishing house operating under the ownership of the European Centre for Governance in Complexity, Kokstadflaten 32, N-5257 Kokstad, Norway. URL: http://www.ecgc.eu

ISBN-13: 987-82-91851-03-7 (e-book)
ISBN-13: 978-82-91851-04-4 (pbk)
https://doi.org/10.24994/2018/b.biomarkers

FOREWORD

Bruce Zetter

Imagine that you were a physician responsible for the treatment of patients with cancer. There are a number of questions that you would like to be able to answer with some degree of certainty. Among these are:

- Is a particular person at greater risk of developing life-threatening cancer than others?
- Which people in the general population actually have cancer?
- When a patient is diagnosed with cancer, what is their prognosis?
- Will removal of the primary tumor (by radiation of surgery) be curative or will it be likely to recur?
- Is there an effective treatment to prevent recurrence?
- Is there a way to detect recurrence in a patient that responded well to treatment?
- If the cancer recurs, is there an effective treatment for that patient's cancer?
- Should the patient be treated with one drug, or with a combination of drugs? If a combination, should the drugs be given at the same time, or one after another?
- Can we predict the amount of toxicity that will affect that patient and does the risk of toxicity outweigh the benefits of the treatment?
- When the patient is being treated, is there a good way to know if the treatment is working, and is there a way to know when it stops working (tumor resistance)? What treatment, if any, should be used next?
- When do we stop treatment and let the patient die gracefully?

Not very long ago, there were almost no tests to provide answers to any of the questions posed above. Progress in the identification of biomarkers over the past 20 years has led to a burgeoning field in which new markers, proposed to answer many of the questions posed above, have been identified and increasingly have proven useful in the clinic. One can anticipate that over the next ten years, tests of various types will emerge that answer most of the above questions. This, however, will not necessarily leave our cancer physicians with a clear path to follow in the treatment and monitoring of their patients. Rather, they will be left with an entirely new set of problems, including:

- Is the test good enough?
- How should the test be interpreted?
- Who will pay for the test?
- If the test indicates a certain treatment, who will pay for that treatment?
- When do we apply "standard of care" and when do we utilize more expensive targeted or immunologic therapies?
- Does the benefit justify the cost? If not, does it make sense to use the biomarker that may indicate the more costly treatment?
- How will we treat patients who cannot afford the best treatments?

Until recently, there have been very few places to obtain the answers to such questions or even to obtain the knowledge that such questions exist, and that thoughtful scientists are giving the thought. To their great credit, Lars Akslen and his colleagues incorporated the study of the ethics and economics of biomarkers into the structure of the CCBIO institute at its inception in 2013. With the expertise of Roger Strand, Anne Blanchard and others, these topics are interwoven into the daily discovery and application of the biomarker research that takes place in the institute. In this volume, they have assembled some of the best thinkers in the field to illuminate these important and complex issues. Those scientists and physicians who read this volume will have a much clearer idea of the place of cancer biomarkers in society and of the broader considerations in applying these tests to the greater population. The book should be required reading for oncologists, medical students, graduate students and especially for those who make policy decisions regarding the use and reimbursement of cancer biomarkers.

PREFACE

Lars A. Akslen

The field of precision medicine is an expanding universe, and galaxies of big data continue to excite basic and clinical scientists. At the same time, there are immediate challenges in how to guide the treatment of cancer patients in the best possible way. The concept of 'targeted therapy and companion biomarkers' needs to be further strengthened with a balance between novel therapy options and linked biomarkers to help navigate modern practice. Transcending the individual patient, there is a need to integrate the fields of ethics and economics and their contributions towards more responsible and just priorities for society.

Biomarker research is an important nexus between basic studies and the range of diagnostic and therapeutic applications. These are continuously discovered from deeper and deeper studies of how malignant tumours function. In their "Hallmarks of Cancer" review paper presented in 2011 (second version), cancer researchers Douglas Hanahan and Robert A. Weinberg established a useful conceptual framework for understanding and communicating different cancer drivers and the intriguing complexity of tumours at the primary and secondary sites – how cancers develop and continue to learn from their surroundings and adapt to new microenvironments after the dissemination phase.

The full clinical potential of biomarkers has not been reached. In particular, their role in novel trial designs should be strengthened. Interactions with the pharmaceutical industry and their policies is a critical issue in this respect. Still, there is an optimistic belief that rapid implementation of new and validated companion biomarkers can 'change the game' of contemporary medical oncology.

Beyond the role of biomarkers in our understanding of cancer biology, additional aspects of biomarker research and use are equally important. When we established and organized the Centre for Cancer Biomarkers (CCBIO), a Norwegian Centre of Excellence, we soon realized that our programs of biological and medical studies needed to be influenced and supported by expertise dealing with economics profiling and the ethics of priority setting.

In this book, important topics surrounding the medical part of biomarker research are presented and discussed. Some key questions are reflected upon: What is a good (enough) biomarker? How should we prioritize in modern cancer treatment? Can biomarkers make a real difference? How can biomarkers change and improve the cost structure when using very expensive drugs and when only a few patients respond to treatment? How can we deal with big and complex data profiles for individual patients – such as patterns of genetic alterations or functional protein signatures?

Hopefully, these thoughtful chapters can stimulate our reflections on how we design and perform biomarker research. On top of basic and clinical studies, we have realized that bringing in these additional research fields have intensified our reflections on our own activities. This goes to the core of the RRI-concept, in other words, to perform responsible research and innovation.

CONTENTS

INTRODUCTION

Anne Blanchard and Roger Strand

Over the last two decades, the field of oncology research and care has been undergoing a shift from a 'one-size-fits all' approach, delivering the same 'blockbuster' drugs to patients with the same cancer, to more personalised cancer medicine. Personalised medicine seeks to address the critiques of the blockbuster model, which has often led to the under- or over-treatment of patients and a concomitant risk of adverse effects. It aims to tailor treatments to sub-groups of patients sharing similar genetic traits and tumour characteristics. One way of personalising cancer treatments is through biomarkers: molecules (like proteins or antibodies) or biochemical changes (like gene expressions and mutations) found in patients' tissue, blood or other body fluids, which indicate the presence of cancer in the body. A metaphor used by Lars Akslen, director of the Centre for Cancer Biomarkers (Bergen, Norway), and author of the preface of this book, depicts cancer biomarkers as the fingerprints of tumours. As fingerprints, they help stratify patients according to their genetics and tumour types, and are used in a clinical setting to help determine predispositions to particular types of cancer, to screen and diagnose cancer types and stages, to estimate the disease prognosis, to predict the most effective course of treatment, and to monitor cancer recurrence.

With all these promises, personalised medicine and cancer biomarkers have received growing attention in the media, increased funding for further

Anne Blanchard and Roger Strand (Eds.), *Cancer Biomarkers: Ethics, Economics and Society.* Bergen: Megaloceros Press, 2017. ISBN 978-82-91851-04-4 (paperback). https://doi.org/10.24994/2018/b.biomarkers © The Authors / Megaloceros Press.

research, and have become priorities of European and American health policies. But research on cancer biomarkers is still relatively new, with only a few biomarkers implemented today in the clinic. Moreover, there is a broad range of scientific, social, ethical and economic issues surrounding this new field, including: how the complexity of cancer biology can impede the robustness of biomarkers in the clinic, the question of national and global justice of prioritising groups of patients or diseases over others, the issue of where to draw the line between the various sub-groups of patients for personalised treatment, or the question of how to evaluate the cost-effectiveness and fairness of personalised cancer treatments. These are all timely issues that are reflected in the existing literature, but that this book aims to address in an assembled way.

This book emerged from cooperation between the various research groups of the Centre for Cancer Biomarkers (CCBIO), looking at the ethical, legal and social aspects of cancer biomarkers, the economic aspects of cancer biomarkers, the prioritisation of health aspects, and the oncology researchers. To add depth to this Norwegian perspective, we also invited two leading scholars on biomarkers and personalised medicine from the United States and Switzerland. By bringing together authors from the fields of science and technology studies, medical ethics and philosophy, priority setting, health economics and oncology, the book aims to give a comprehensive and critical overview of some of the key social, ethical and economic issues that surround cancer biomarkers. At the same time, we have strived to create a volume that is accessible to a wide audience ranging from researchers to practitioners and decision-makers at large in the field of personalised medicine.

First in this volume, Chapter 1 (by Anne Blanchard and Elisabeth Wik) sets the scene for the discussion of the various social, ethical and economic aspects around biomarkers by interrogating the notion of a 'good enough' biomarker in the context of the high complexity and uncertainties around the biology of cancer, and of limited health care resources. After defining biomarkers and their different purposes, the chapter explores the 'ideal' attributes that a biomarker should have from a medical and a health policy point of view. In brief, an ideal biomarker should altogether demonstrate analytical validity, clinical validity and clinical utility, while contributing to the sustainability of health care systems and remaining accessible to patients nationally and globally. Arguably, these expectations are very hard to meet. This is why the authors introduce the concept of 'good enough' biomarkers, where their sophistication and quality depends on their purpose. Good enough biomarkers could help reintroduce some human judgement into discussions of what we want from cancer research and care, when faced with rich biological and social complexities.

Chapter 2 (by Mikyung Kelly Seo) moves on to look at assessing the economic value of cancer biomarkers, when these do not directly contribute to quality-adjusted life years or mortality in patients. Even if there are a number of studies evaluating the economic costs of various biomarkers for personalised therapies, there is still no clear evaluation of the benefit of biomarkers in economic terms. The chapter addresses some of the challenges of such economic evaluations, ranging from the absence of clear and harmonised guidelines for evaluating the cost-effectiveness of biomarkers, to the problem of comparing economic evaluations across different biomarkers, and the issue of how best to design clinical trials and measure health outcomes of personalised therapies. The author argues that clear guidelines assessing the cost-effectiveness of cancer biomarkers are needed for their timely integration into clinical routines.

Chapter 3 (by John Cairns) follows up on these arguments by looking at how cancer biomarkers can challenge the economic evaluation of targeted cancer therapies, as we move from broad groups of patients to increasingly smaller sub-groups. This is illustrated by economic evaluations of different treatments for non-small cell lung cancer (NSCLC). The challenges of evaluating the treatment costs and effectiveness for NSCLC relate to the difficulties of modelling the effect of a treatment over time and on a representative patient population, to estimate the quality of life gained by different treatment options (in particular to attribute values to the different health states – progression-free, progressed disease and death – the patients spend time in), and to evaluate the quantity of each drug which would be used in the different treatment options. The author concludes that cancer biomarkers may bring greater challenges to the economic evaluation of targeted therapies, because the treatments are more stratified, and therefore estimating clinical effectiveness and cost-effectiveness may be more difficult.

With the issues around the evaluation of cancer biomarkers in mind, Chapter 4 (by Eirik Tranvåg and Ole Frithjof Norheim) bridges economic and ethical issues by looking at how biomarkers influence health resource allocation and priority setting for cancer drugs. The recent approval of the biomarker PD-L1 for treatment of advanced non-squamous cell lung cancer (NSCLC) is used as an example to illustrate how biomarkers can influence priority setting in Norway. After presenting a framework of general principles for health care priority setting, the authors discuss how biomarkers can potentially influence three key criteria for priority setting: (i) the health-benefit criterion, whereby priority is given to a medical intervention that increases the health benefits for the patient; (ii) the resource criterion, according to which priority is given to an intervention that does not require much in terms of resources and is easily implemented in the clinic; and (iii) the severity criterion, when priority is given to an intervention that addresses severe conditions. The authors conclude that

PD-L1 helps guide priority decisions for the first two criteria, as this biomarker indicates patient populations that will most benefit from a treatment for NSCLC, and points to treatments that will necessitate less in terms of resources for their implementation in a clinical setting. The potential of PD-L1 for guiding priority decisions according to the severity criterion for treatment of NSCLC is less clear.

Following these reflections on health care priority setting and the fair allocation of resources in Norway, Chapter 5 (by Leonard M. Fleck) brings the ethical debates around health care justice and rationing to the American context. This chapter is illustrative of the difficult intersection between the ethics, economics and politics of expensive cancer drugs and their biomarkers, and addresses several related points. It discusses the fair distribution of personalised treatments, which should not be restricted to well-insured and wealthy groups of patients. It further looks at the issue of 'ragged edges' and the absence of a clear line between respondents and non-respondents to cancer therapies, which complicate this fair allocation of treatments. The author also interrogates whether the successes of cancer biomarkers are replicable, and what we should do in the case where only a small proportion of patients with the same biomarker might respond to a personalised treatment. Finally, the author discusses the case of 'super-responders', and whether they should be the only ones having access to expensive targeted treatments. This is discussed in broader terms that link back to Chapters 2 and 3: does cost-effectiveness actually matter in questions of health care resource allocation? In a short epilogue, written shortly before the book went into print, Fleck also provides a comment to the possible consequences of the change in administration in the US in 2017. The epilogue was written before the so-called Obamacare survived the first attempt of "repeal and replace" in March 2017, but its bleak forecast of what might take place in the near future remains timely and relevant.

Chapter 6 (by Alessandro Blasimme) continues to explore ethical questions around cancer biomarkers, and in particular the ethical issues emerging with a 'big data' or multiplex-data approach to personalised medicine, that builds on a wide variety of patient data (genome sequences, 'omics' data, etc.). In his chapter, the author employs the theoretical framework of "co-production", showing how the imaginary of personalised medicine at the same time is a matter of crafting future promises and policies of science, health care and health politics. Interestingly, the political agenda of personalised medicine that emerged in the US embraces ideas of inclusion and empowerment of the individual citizen-patient; if and how this can be translated into practice remains, however, an unsettled question.

Part of that settlement will depend on how we as individuals and as a civilisation come to terms with the underlying existential issues of suffering

4

and fear of death as technological barriers continue to be pushed and moved.

Chapter 7 (by Caroline Engen) introduces broader reflections on how personalised cancer medicine might influence the care-cure relationship, in particular relative to over-diagnosis, over-treatment and greater medicalisation. The author argues that cancer biomarkers and their promise for guiding precise and targeted therapies might lead to an increasingly fragmented vision and understanding of cancer, as well as to a greater hope of controlling this disease. The author thus points to the need to design realistic goals for cancer research and care while facing the eternal questions about our own existence, including our own certain mortality.

Finally, Chapter 8 (by Roger Strand) tries to summarise some of the contentious issues around expensive cancer drugs and explores what a post-normal framing of personalised medicine can offer to address the distrust between cancer patients and the institutional and scientific logic that prioritise the sustainability of health care systems. "Post-normal" problems are defined as problems in which a lot is at stake, decisions are urgent, facts may be uncertain and values are in dispute. In such situations, the chapter argues, scientific and institutional improvements are of course valuable but the general problem of distrust cannot be expected to go away easily. Regarding other such issues, typically revolving around environmental or technological risk, scholars have proposed means to create more inclusive and democratic forms of decision-making and governance. Could that work for the contentious issues around cancer, and what role might biomarkers play?

In one sense, then, the volume as such makes a full circle. It begins with the seemingly simple and innocent question of what constitutes a "good" biomarker before it delves into the complex issues of ethics, economics, institutions, politics and the existential background onto which, adding metaphor onto metaphor, "battles" over the "War on Cancer" are fought. The seemingly simple question about the good biomarker is entangled into questions about the Good (caring and just) Society, the future of Science and ultimately the Good Life. The theoretical framework of post-normal science has been a strong source of inspiration throughout the academic work of we who have edited this volume. The first tenet of post-normal science, when attending to questions about Quality, be it of science, medicine or life, would be to ask: Quality for whom? Judged by whom? With this volume we offer an interdisciplinary response to the questions of quality. It is our hope that the ideas in this book will inspire and provoke our readers to respond and contribute to what we believe are important discussions about the future of cancer research and cancer care. It seems appropriate to end this introduction with the words of ASCO, the American Society of Clinical Oncology, who in their vision document

Shaping the Future of Oncology: Envisioning Cancer Care in 2030, stated: "By anticipating the future, we can shape it."

The publication of this book would not have been possible without the continuous effort and support of a large number of friends and colleagues. First and foremost we thank our co-authors who delivered in every sense of the word, including complying with our ambitious time schedule. We are most grateful to Idun Strand Hauge and Emma Hjellestad for excellent copy-editing and design services, respectively. CCBIO, notably its Director Lars A. Akslen, Project Manager Geir Olav Løken and its Scientific Advisory Board, and the Centre for the Study of the Sciences and the Humanities (University of Bergen) provided financial and moral support throughout the book project. Most of the research presented in the individual chapters was funded by the Research Council of Norway through CCBIO's Centre of Excellence grant. Finally, publishing together with the European Centre for Governance in Complexity and its Megaloceros Press made it possible to produce an affordable but high quality publication in a fraction of the time that many conventional publishing houses require.

1

WHAT IS A GOOD (ENOUGH) BIOMARKER?

Anne Blanchard and Elisabeth Wik

1. Introduction: The hype around personalised medicine and cancer biomarkers

Personalised cancer medicine is a priority in European policies shaping future cancer research and care. These policies come on the back of recent developments in 'omics' technologies that look into cancer at a molecular level to identify new biomarkers. Last year, the European Commission claimed: "Personalised medicine is an interdisciplinary field that will drive the health research and innovation agenda for years to come." (EC, 2016a; p. 1) This optimism has seen important financial support allocated to encourage the development of personalised medicine, first through the European Seventh Framework Programme for research and innovation, where the EU dedicated over €1 billion for this research between 2007-2013, and now through the Horizon 2020 Framework Programme, with €50 million dedicated to the field in 2016. Similarly, funding for research and development of personalised cancer medicine is one of the priorities in Norwegian health policies, with the Ministry of Health and Care Services dedicating a budget of 8 million NOK (about €900,000) for the year 2017 alone (Helsedirektoratet, 2016; HOD, 2016).

In these policy documents, personalised medicine is about "tailoring the right therapeutic strategy for the right person at the right time, and/or to

Anne Blanchard and Roger Strand (Eds.), *Cancer Biomarkers: Ethics, Economics and Society*. Bergen: Megaloceros Press, 2017. ISBN 978-82-91851-04-4 (paperback). https://doi.org/10.24994/2018/b.biomarkers © The Authors / Megaloceros Press.

determine the predisposition to disease, and/or to deliver timely and targeted prevention" (EC, 2015; p. 3). In this context, biomarkers play an important role as "quantifiable parameters predictive of the development of a disease, disease prognosis [...] or targets for new treatments" (EC, 2013; p. 6).

But what is a biomarker? In 1998, the American National Institute of Health's working group on biomarkers defined a biomarker as a "characteristic that is objectively measured and evaluated as an indicator of normal biologic processes, pathogenic processes, or pharmacologic responses to a therapeutic intervention" (NIH, 2001). Cancer biomarkers support decisions related to diagnosis and treatment with three main purposes, defining: who to treat (prognostic markers); how to treat (predictive markers); and how much to treat (pharmacodynamic markers), as illustrated by Figure 1.

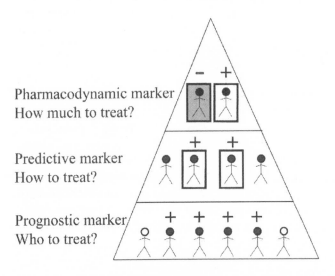

Figure 1. The three main purposes of cancer biomarkers for prognostication and therapy decisions. Reading from the base to the top of the pyramid, '+' means that the patient is 'marker positive' and goes to the next level of biomarker assessment. '+' and '–' at the top of the pyramid means adjustment of the dosage of medicine given. (Figure by E. Wik.)

Cancer biomarkers are markers that may relate to the eight proposed hallmarks that characterise cancer; ranging from limitless replicative potential of the cells, to sustained angiogenesis (blood vessels that vascularise and 'feed' the tumour), and to tissue invasion and metastasis (for the extensive list, see Hanahan and Weinberg, 2011). These distinctive features of cancer are caused by a broad range of genetic and epigenetic aberrations as well as by dysregulated communication between cancer cells themselves, and between cancer cells and cells in the surrounding tumour microenvironment. To better understand these cancer hallmarks and the biologic processes taking place within and between the cells of a tumour, cancer biomarkers have been a focus of research for more than half a century. Today, biomarkers play an important role when searching for new therapeutic approaches or strategies in cancer treatment, and they are considered crucial to the improvement of personalised medicine (Vargas and Harris, 2016).

Going deeper into the three main purposes of biomarkers, *prognostic biomarkers* identify groups among cancer patients that are likely to experience recurrence and shorter survival due to their disease. These patient groups may potentially benefit from more extensive therapy to reduce the risk of recurrent disease, and to improve their survival if the treatment is effective. Prognostic biomarkers can also help identify patients that may experience long survival with less therapy, and thus spare them the potentially severe side effects of therapies that would not be needed in their case. In endometrial cancer for instance, morphologic measures like histologic grade (measure of the degree to which the tumour looks like the normal tissue from where it originated: grade 1 to 3) and the depth of myometrial invasion (the proportion of the muscle layer in the uterus that is invaded by tumour tissues) are examples of prognostic markers (Salvesen et al., 2012). *Predictive biomarkers* predict the patient's response to a specific therapy. For breast cancer for instance, the oestrogen receptor and HER2 status are functioning both as part of a panel of prognostic markers, and as predictive markers, by directing hormone therapy and anti-HER2 therapy to breast cancer patients (Early Breast Cancer Trialists' Collaborative et al., 2011; Slamon et al., 2011). When the appropriate drug for the appropriate patient is selected, *pharmacodynamic biomarkers* may further assist in selecting the optimal dose at which the drug should be administered to the patient to improve the efficiency of the treatment and reduce side effects (Ventola, 2013). One example of a pharmacodynamic marker is the variation in a single nucleotide (single nucleotide polymorphism, SNP) of the gene *NRG3*, indicating increased responsiveness to platinum therapeutics in ovarian cancer (Ni et al., 2013). However, the study of pharmacodynamic cancer biomarkers is an emerging field, with no such biomarkers yet approved by the American Food and Drug Administration.

Relative to these three purposes, the main types of applied prognostic and predictive cancer biomarkers are: (i) *clinical markers* like blood pressure (Schuster et al., 2012) and surgical staging (identifying the spread of cancer, especially for ovarian cancer); (ii) *histopathologic markers* like tumour size and histologic grade in breast and endometrial carcinomas; (iii) *molecular markers* like the specific EGFR and KRAS mutations in lung and colorectal cancer, and HER2 gene amplification and/or protein expression in breast cancer; and more recently, (iv) *imaging biomarkers* which could, through radiologic images, help in the preoperative work-up to tailor the surgical therapy that is offered to the patient (Salvesen et al., 2012).

Cancer biomarkers are promising tools in support of personalised medicine. However, the complexity, plurality and uncertainties around the mechanisms of cancer should make us cautious when biomarkers are depicted as able to allow both comprehensive and robust insights into cancer, and better, safer and economically sustainable medical decision-making and therapies. In this chapter, co-authored by ELSA (Ethical, Legal and Social Aspects of cancer biomarkers) researcher Anne Blanchard and breast cancer researcher Elisabeth Wik, we interrogate widespread notions of what constitutes an 'ideal' cancer biomarker; one that is sophisticated enough to solve both biological questions and ethical dilemmas. In this way, the chapter offers a novel contribution that is both *integrative* of different biological and social aspects of biomarkers, and *critical* of the image portrayed in the oncology literature and in most policy documents.

Section 2 looks at the ideal cancer biomarker as pictured in the oncology literature, where biomarkers are usually praised for their accuracy, precision, sensitivity, specificity, safety for the patient and their simplicity. Then, Section 3 looks at the ideal biomarker as described in recent European policy documents, whereby biomarkers are expected to help guide better-informed medical decisions, improve the health and quality of life of cancer patients, contribute to the sustainability of health care systems, while ensuring fair accessibility to personalised medicine both nationally and globally. In Section 4, we discuss the key questions that come to challenge 'ideal' biomarkers in the face of rich biological, social, ethical and economic complexities, and introduce the notion of 'good enough' biomarkers as a way to more constructively reflect on these complexities and uncertainties. Finally, in Section 5, we conclude that cancer biomarkers that leave room for debating social and ethical questions in a context of personalised medicine are indeed 'good enough', and make important contributions to the research and care in a context of personalised cancer medicine.

2. The 'ideal' biomarker from the oncology perspective

In oncology, a biomarker is usually praised for its accuracy, precision, sensitivity, specificity, safety for the patient, and also for its simplicity. In biomarker development, from discovery to clinical use, there are however multiple steps to overcome before a biomarker test is approved for clinical application; among them the challenges relating to the reproducibility and validation of the research (see for instance Blanchard, 2016). The oncology literature recognises three broad criteria of a good biomarker.

First, a robust biomarker test should demonstrate *analytical validity*; a concept that encompasses reproducibility, sensitivity, specificity and ease to perform. It is mandatory, in the development of a biomarker, to have a biomarker test assay that reliably reflects the biomarker under study, not only in the research setting but also in routine laboratory practice. In this way, the test assay should reliably measure what it is expected to measure, with a high degree of accuracy and precision; allowing for the assay to be reproduced and validated. The test's sensitivity and specificity also need to be demonstrated. The sensitivity indicates the biomarker's ability to correctly identify patients with the disease, while the specificity indicates the biomarker's ability to correctly identify patients without the disease (Freidlin et al., 2012). An increase in sensitivity is gained at the expense of specificity, and vice versa. Therefore, a test assay having both full sensitivity and specificity is impossible to achieve (Füzéry et al., 2013), and the balance between sensitivity and specificity needs to be reached according to the purpose of the biomarker. In addition, the test should be relatively easy to perform in routine laboratory practice and in subsequent clinical practice.

Second, the biomarker test has to demonstrate *clinical validity*, meaning that it can identify defined end-points of interest, for instance patients at risk of recurrent disease, in independent patient cohorts. The biomarker should therefore be able to separate cancer patients into two groups with different outcomes, like responders versus non-responders to a specific therapy, or healthy survivors versus patients at risk of early death due to cancer (Teutsch et al., 2009). Defining relevant cut-off levels of the biomarker test is extremely important (Majewski and Bernards, 2011; Gutman and Kessler, 2006; Vargas and Harris, 2016), as it has major impacts for the patients who might be granted (or not) a particular therapy according to their test results.

Third, the biomarker test should demonstrate *clinical utility*: does it improve patients' outcomes compared with current patient management without the test? (Teutsch et al., 2009) This is often difficult to evaluate, and retrospective studies require large numbers of samples that reflect the heterogeneity of the target population, to examine if a biomarker test is of real clinical interest. In order to evaluate clinical utility, the last phase of biomarker development generally consists in a randomised clinical trial, where the biomarker is included as part of an algorithm allocating patients to therapy A or therapy B, depending on the test (Mordente et al., 2015). But it has been a challenge to standardise such trials and perform comparative validation studies, and ideally multicentre studies should be carried out as part of the test validation phase. In addition, the standard set-up of clinical trials, with a prospective and randomised design, is costly and time-consuming, and must these days give way to other more dynamic and adaptive study designs.

With all these steps from biomarker discovery to clinical use, only very few biomarkers have reached clinical practice (Diamandis, 2012; Kern, 2012). There are nevertheless biomarkers that are now considered 'a success', like the marker HER2, a gene and protein biomarker that is today used in clinical practice for breast cancer patients. The development and story of HER2 as a prognostic marker, a target for therapy and a predictive marker for the anti-HER2 therapy, unfolded over 20 years. It started in 1984 when Weinberg and colleagues identified the human epidermal growth factor receptor 2 gene (*HER2/neu* gene) (Schechter et al., 1984), and in 1998, the first version of the HER2 therapy/biomarker package was completed. The Food and Drug Administration (FDA) went on to approve trastuzumab (a monoclonal antibody directed towards HER2) as therapy to breast cancer patients with advanced tumours showing HER2 amplification and/or overexpressing the HER2 protein (Ross et al., 2009). However, there is a side-story to the success of HER2 in breast cancer. Primary resistance to trastuzumab has been observed in patients with HER2 amplified tumours, indicating that the tumour biology is not as simple as to expect cure and no recurrence by simply inhibiting one tumour protein. Therefore, combinatorial therapies including trastuzumab and HER2 diagnostic testing have been explored (Ross et al., 2009; Swain et al., 2015; Krop et al., 2014; Verma et al., 2012), and several therapy combinations are now approved by the FDA and EMA (European Medicines Agency). These are either as treatment of metastatic breast cancer or as adjuvant therapy (therapy given in addition to the primary surgery, to prevent recurrent disease) to breast cancer patients. This side-story of HER2 is interesting as it points to the complexity of coming up with 'ideal' biomarkers for a disease as complex and uncertain as cancer.

3. The 'ideal' biomarker from the health policy perspective

Echoing expectations towards biomarkers found in the oncology literature, recent European and Norwegian health policy documents also see personalised medicine as a priority for cancer research and care, with biomarkers anticipated to fulfil many promises. According to these documents, the 'ideal' biomarker should be able to: (i) help make better-informed medical decisions; (ii) improve the health and quality of life of cancer patients; (iii) contribute to the sustainability of health care systems; and (iv) have fair and just accessibility both nationally and globally.

First, *better-informed medical decisions* are expected through personalised medicine as it "tailor[s] the right therapeutic strategy for the right person at the right time" (EC, 2015; p. 3); providing the "ability to make more informed medical decisions" (EC, 2013; p. 5). Indeed, as seen in the introduction, having a relevant cancer biomarker helps medical practitioners choose between various treatment options, doses, frequency and timing of the treatment, to ensure that the therapy is fitted to the needs of the patients and corresponds to their genetic make-up and tumour characteristics. Another dimension of better-informed medical decisions is the 'patient-centred' focus of personalised medicine, in order that "greater participation by patients in the management of their own health [will] help prevent disease and promote healthy living" (EC, 2016b; p. 5). Patient-centred medicine means encouraging the "active participation of the patients in decision-making processes concerning their treatment" (Helsedirektoratet, 2016; p. 5), with the goal of enhancing the quality and safety of care for each patient (EC, 2015). It also means that patients will be further involved in "the formulation of treatment guidelines and protocols, the design of clinical trials and medicine reimbursement" (EU, 2016b; p. 5), to discuss how targeted therapies can be distributed equitably among patients who need them.

Second, and related to the previous point, personalised medicine and cancer biomarkers are anticipated to *improve the health and quality of life of cancer patients* by offering better-targeted treatments that reduce "adverse reactions to medicinal products" that are too strongly or too weakly dosed for the patient (EC, 2015; p. 3). In addition, because some biomarkers focus on the prevention and prediction of disease, they can help determine peoples' predisposition to certain types of cancer and allow "earlier disease intervention than has been possible in the past" (EC, 2013; p. 5). As emphasised by the European Commission, "the identification of multiple biomarkers [...] could make it possible to use detailed risk profiling as an additional tool for targeted interventions, aiming at and potentially improving health outcomes" (EC, 2015; p. 3).

Third, European policy documents raise the concern that public budget deficits and an ageing population are putting public health budgets under considerable strain: "ever-increasing resources are required to treat diseases such as cancers, chronic or degenerative diseases and diabetes" (EC, 2013; p. 24). In this context, cancer biomarkers are expected to "*contribute to addressing the sustainability of healthcare systems*" (EC, 2015; p. 2) and "improve health care cost containment" (EC, 2013; p. 5). The rationale behind this is that personalised medicine will in one way help allocate better-targeted treatments that will limit side-effects of too high toxicity therapies, and the resulting snowballing medicalisation to treat these side-effects; and in another way, through a focus on prevention and early disease detection, will bring treatment costs down (EC, 2016b), and allow "over time [...] for a more cost-efficient use of healthcare" (EU, 2015; p. 3).

Finally, targeted therapies offered by personalised medicine are significantly more expensive than the standard 'blockbuster' drugs proposed to patients suffering from the same cancer type, without distinction of genetic make-up or tumour characteristics. An important point in policy documents is that these targeted treatments *should remain accessible to all, both nationally and globally*, with for instance the Norwegian Directorate of Health claiming: "Personalised medicine uses emergent technology-based approaches and is highly specialised. The implementation of personalised medicine requires an approach that can ensure that these interventions are equitable and available for patients in all regions of the country." (Helsedirektoratet, 2016; p. 5) Accordingly, 'patient-centred' healthcare where patients are active in designing their own treatment options, but also the institutional and reimbursement frameworks of personalised medicine, will help ensuring the fair distribution of healthcare products and services. But would that really be enough? Expectations towards cancer biomarkers in policy documents are very high, and can be easily challenged by the complexity of cancer and the complexity of the socio-economic systems where personalised medicine is nested, as discussed in Section 4 below.

4. Discussion: going from 'ideal' to 'good enough' biomarkers?

Sections 2 and 3 showed how cancer biomarkers can be described in an 'ideal' way, allowing for both robust insights into the complex biology of cancer, and better, safer and economically sustainable medical decision-making. However, even if cancer biomarkers are promising tools for designing and allocating better-targeted therapies, the biological and clinical reality of cancer remains complex and uncertain, making it difficult to design an 'ideal' biomarker. Indeed, dividing cancer patients into subgroups of strong, weak or non-responders to a particular therapy is not straightforward, and Fleck (2012) argues that the clinical reality in metastatic cancer is most often a continuum of responses from weak to strong. The heterogeneity characterising cancer (within a single tumour, but also within different tumours in the same patient, and between patients), as well as technical aspects in laboratory work (such as a lack of standardised methods across laboratories, and challenges of reproducibility and validation), make it difficult to come up with an ideal biomarker that finds relevant application in the clinical setting.

In this section, we turn to some of the key questions that come to challenge this idea of 'ideal' biomarkers portrayed in the oncology literature and in policy documents, and we argue for introducing the more humble notion of 'good enough' cancer biomarkers in oncology research and political and social discourses, as a more constructive way to look at the rich biological and social complexities around cancer.

a. To match the complexity of cancer biology, should a biomarker be equally complex and composite?

Intra-tumour heterogeneity (i.e., heterogeneity within a tumour) is recognised as deserving more attention for better understanding cancer biology and for improving personalised medicine (Gerlinger et al., 2012; Vargas and Harris, 2016). Varying expression of genes and proteins within the different cellular parts of the tumour, and within different areas of the tumour, has been a scientific challenge for researchers aiming to identify targets for therapy and the accompanying therapeutics, and for the development of robust cancer biomarkers. What does it mean, in terms of test validity, if the expression of biomarker 'A' varies greatly within different areas of the tumour? The patient may get the result 'A positive' or 'A negative', depending on where in the tumour the sample is taken (see Figure 2). And if the protein 'A' is also a target for therapy, the consequences for the patients are tremendous as they are offered or denied a therapy according to their test results.

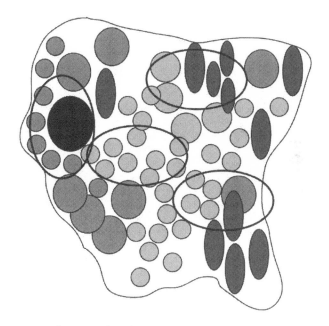

Figure 2. Intra-tumour heterogeneity: The figure illustrates a tumour composed of various elements and their expression (different coloured and sized dots, respectively) in different areas of the tumour. The black elliptical circles represent different areas of tissue sampling for the biomarker test. One-molecule biomarkers will focus on the presence of one particular element in the sampling area (even if several elements are present in this area); while composite biomarkers (calculating the sum of expression of the various molecules) are able to pick up on different elements simultaneously, giving a more robust test result that is more representative of the intra-tumour heterogeneity. (Figure by E. Wik.)

So how can intra-tumour heterogeneity be addressed by biomarkers? As seen in Section 2, the observation of primary trastuzumab resistance in breast cancer patients with HER2 positive tumours shows that cancer biology is complex, and that targeting only one specific tumour alteration is often insufficient for achieving tumour reduction or cure. It indeed seems reasonable to assume that single molecules cannot alone initiate, drive and sustain tumour growth. On this basis more complex biomarker panels, also called signature or *composite biomarkers*, are put forward to compensate for the lack of knowledge regarding 'the complete picture' of specific signalling pathways and their de-regulation (see Figure 2). Gene expression (mRNA) microarrays were amongst the first methods where data covering the whole genome was included in the search for composite cancer biomarkers (Golub et al., 1999). A few landmark publications in the microarray field set the standard for a new way of thinking about cancer biomarkers (Alizadeh et al., 2000; Perou et al., 2000). Researchers argued that, compared to the detection of single gene alterations, global scale data may have a greater potential for reflecting intra-tumour heterogeneity, and for identifying markers for more complex biological processes taking place in the cancer cells. Such gene expression arrays have been increasingly applied in translational cancer research in the past 20 years. In addition to identifying both known and new molecular phenotypes in various cancer types – such as breast, bladder and colorectal cancer – composite biomarkers have proven to be reliable in predicting cancer recurrences in breast and colorectal cancer (van't Veer et al., 2002; Li et al., 2012), and in identifying relevant targets for therapy (Rouzier et al., 2005) along with markers predicting response to specific treatment regimens (Loi et al., 2013; Oshima et al., 2011).

Now, with the emergence of new 'omics' approaches, it is possible to go beyond the levels of single genes and proteins, and cover large-scale data at different biological levels (e.g. DNA, epigenetic molecules, metabolites). On the basis of these new approaches, collaborative initiatives such as the Cancer Genome Atlas Network aim to gather together multiple levels of 'omics' data from large populations and for many cancer types (*https://cancergenome.nih.gov/*). This 'multi-level omics approach' has led to new cancer subclasses, defined by composite biomarkers composed of different types of molecules (TCGA Network, 2012; Cancer Genome Atlas Research et al., 2013). Recent publications show that cancer research is further developing in the direction of composite biomarkers: in a review on biomarker development in lung cancer, Vargas and Harris (2016) propose to combine data from the genome, the transcriptome, the epigenome, the microbiome, and the metabolome, along with information from the exposome, epidemiologic data and clinical information, into knowledge networks that will potentially give new taxonomic classifications to disease panels. This approach is also supported by European health policies, with the Commission arguing that "for the development of stratification biomarkers [a] multiple approach integrating various technologies ('omics', phenotype studies, imaging, functional *in vivo* studies, etc.) needs to be pursued" (EC, 2013; p. 10).

But do these sophisticated composite biomarkers really help address intra-tumour heterogeneity? By measuring various tumour elements, at various biological levels, composite biomarkers might indeed reflect a larger proportion of all the mechanisms driving and sustaining tumour growth and disease progress. However, compared to one-molecule biomarkers, composite biomarkers raise a number of issues, both at the oncology and socio-economic levels. First, when developing a composite biomarker, there is an increased risk of false positive test results, because of testing multiple markers at the same time. Appropriate study design and cohort selection in validation studies are important to reduce this risk, even though the risk itself will always remain (Polley et al., 2013). Beyond the stress and discomfort caused to the patients by a greater risk of false positive results, it seems that results from these sophisticated tests cannot be displayed without consideration for the ambiguities and uncertainties surrounding them. This makes the subsequent medical decision-making less straightforward and could lead to an increase in costs if the appropriate therapy is not found promptly after the test. Second, and related to the previous point, even a sophisticated composite biomarker cannot disclose everything. These tests can only look at a limited number of tumour elements, when countless factors actually enter into play in the development of a cancer tumour. Arguably, even composite biomarkers have what Fredriksen (2006; p. 452) calls 'a tunnel vision': "they highlight only a small spot of the possible field of investigation". Further investigations are thus often needed, resulting in a 'snowballing medicalisation' and increased costs (Fredriksen, 2006). Third, when developing composite biomarkers, the weaknesses and biases inherent to the exploration of one-molecule biomarkers are amplified when including various tissue types and various techniques for extracting and measuring different molecules, and up-scaling the multiple testing in analyses of 'omics' data. This poses the question of how far we can and should go in the 'sophistication' of biomarkers, if the results are in the end still (and arguably more) uncertain and ambiguous. This is further discussed in Section 4.d.

In sum, even if composite biomarkers better reflect the various mechanisms that come into play in tumour growth and disease progression, and even if they have already allowed important insights and discoveries in cancer biology, the more sophisticated a biomarker is, the more it seems to face stringent challenges of quality, validation and ease to implement in a clinical setting.

b.   To better understand the evolutive nature of cancer, should a biomarker be measured sequentially over time?

Tumour cell evolution seems to follow a 'survival of the fittest' rule, and targeting cancerous cells is analogous to shooting at a moving target. What then can we actually expect from cancer biomarker tests, when these are mere snapshots of the tumour at one point in time, and only give a static representation of the disease?

To address the evolutive nature of cancer, a more dynamic approach in biomarker development has been to do *sequential measurements* – measurements of biomarkers done at different points in time – either in solid tumours or in circulating tumour cells (CTCs). CTCs are found in the patient's blood after having been shed into the vasculature from the primary tumour. The CTCs are potential seeds for metastatic cancer, and thus potential markers for recurrent disease. Both the presence and quantification of CTCs in blood samples, as well as proteins and genomic alterations in the CTCs themselves, are explored as potential cancer biomarkers (Nakazawa et al., 2015; Qi and Wang, 2016). Sequential measurements of CTCs would give a more dynamic picture of the evolution of the disease, and measuring these biomarkers throughout a therapy for instance, would provide some insights into tumour cell evolution, with potential benefits for the patients as therapy could then be readjusted over time. Let us consider a patient with a HER2 negative primary tumour, who receives chemotherapy for her advanced, metastatic disease. After a few rounds of this therapy regimen, a biopsy of a metastatic lesion is found to be HER2 positive. In this case, the patient could receive a readjusted, anti-HER2 medication.

While sequential biomarker measurements show promise, there are a number of issues raised by this dynamic approach to sampling biomarkers. First, from the patient's perspective, sequential biomarker measurements mean that they have to undergo tests more regularly. While it can be reassuring for some patients, it can also be a source of stress due to the potential invasive nature of these tests (such as surgical biopsies of solid tumours), the waiting time for results, or, in the case of CTCs, the uncertainty around whether there are sufficient tumour cells present in the blood to justify further therapy. Indeed, what does it mean to have three tumour cells in the blood, and what is the threshold for further therapy? This is scientifically still unclear. Second, it is debatable whether it is actually beneficial for the patient to constantly receive new drugs during the course of a therapy, with varying mechanisms of action and the various side effects they have to adapt to. Finally, sequential biomarker measurements pose the question of their implementation in the clinic and of generating additional costs. Taking several biomarker measurements over time for each patient presupposes more manpower for making these measurements and analysing the results. This arguably has the consequence of raising the overall cost of the therapy for the patient; negating any benefit of biomarkers for the sustainability of health care systems. It might also go against the equitable and fair accessibility of such 'hyper-personalised' treatments, that are tailored not only to the patient's initial tumour characteristics, but over time to his/her changing needs. This question of economic sustainability is discussed in Section 4c below.

c. *Is it possible to have a cancer biomarker that is sophisticated, as well as economically sustainable and widely accessible?*

Composite biomarkers and biomarkers that are measured sequentially over time bring key insights into the biology of cancer. However, can such sophisticated biomarkers also be economically sustainable and widely accessible to patients? According to European policy documents, public health budgets are already under considerable strain (EC, 2013). In this context, personalised medicine, in particular for cancer, is expected to help cut costs relative to over-treatment: "The French Cancer Institute has shown that investing in molecular testing for the use of stratified and targeted medicines can in fact bring significant savings to the public health sector, as the cost of testing is offset by the reduction in non-effective or inappropriate prescribing." (EC, 2013; p. 24-25) However, as discussed in Chapters 2 and 3 of this book, evaluating the cost-effectiveness of cancer biomarkers is difficult, and there are very few existing studies trying to address whether the cost of diagnostic tests counterbalances the prescription of inappropriate therapies. Whether cancer biomarkers are contributing to the sustainability of health care systems remains an open question, and even more so for sophisticated biomarkers, as the advanced technologies they rely on induce supplementary costs for their implementation in the clinic. Another consideration is that even if we might be able to analyse complex biomarkers at a lower cost than at present, it might nonetheless encourage the use of complex biomarker technology; as a step towards ramping up aggregated costs.

Regarding the question of social justice and fair and equitable access to personalised cancer therapies, the Norwegian Ministry of Health and Care Services suggests the following: "Implementation of personalised medicine should be based on established criteria for priority setting in healthcare and should be socio-economically sustainable." (Helsedirektoratet, 2016; p. 6) Are these priority settings enough, however, to ensure fair access to personalised medicine? If some personalised cancer treatments are prioritised, what will they come at the expense of? Personalised medicine can potentially add billions of euros per year to the cost of public health care in Europe, and this burden will need to be met by increased taxes or privatisation through the insurance sector (Blanchard, 2016). As Jackson and Sood (2011) argue, insurers facing these costs in the USA have begun off-loading the expenses onto patients, with an estimated of 62% of all personal bankruptcies attributable to medical costs, principally related to cancer. This issue is even more salient with sophisticated biomarkers. Although it can be argued that the advanced technologies (such as next generation sequencing) on which sophisticated biomarkers rely will to some extent see their cost decrease over time, these technologies remain demanding when it comes to performance in a routine laboratory. Many of the newer, more sophisticated tests already on the market require fresh tissue samples, handled in specific manners to avoid the degradation of the molecules. This of course has implications for accessibility for laboratories in low-income countries, where formalin-fixed paraffin-embedded tissues (i.e., tissue samples that are not 'fresh', but sliced, fixed in formalin, and kept in blocks of paraffin, and thus demand less constraining storage infrastructure) are at the moment the only type of sample they can work on, for economic reasons. Under these conditions, personalised cancer medicine is likely to remain accessible mainly to wealthy and well-insured patients.

d. What then is a 'good enough' biomarker?

Considering the difficulty to have an 'ideal' biomarker that is at the same time sophisticated, easily implemented in the clinical setting, widely accessible and economically sustainable, we can question the orientation of research on cancer biomarkers, that gives increasingly more attention to complex, sophisticated biomarkers. Why not also invest research time on simpler biomarkers, which would not have a very high sensitivity and specificity, but would still deliver acceptable results at a much lower cost? For instance, instead of sequential biomarker measurements and composite biomarkers, why not rather do simple tests on samples from paraffin blocks, or on one immune-marker rather than on a hundred? Studies have shown that there are ways to simplify the extreme complexity that is seen in recent research (like studies from The Cancer Genome Atlas Network merging all 'omics' levels into composite biomarkers), without losing too much in quality. Cuzick et al. (2011) demonstrated that combining four immunohistochemistry biomarkers, assessed on paraffin-embedded tissues, gave a prognostic value similar to an FDA approved multi-genomic test. These tests could be accessible and applicable in laboratories worldwide.

The choice between simple or sophisticated biomarkers depends on the research purpose: is the biomarker's main objective to help us better understand the complexity of cancer – in which case sophisticated biomarkers might be better suited; or is it to have a strong clinical utility and widespread accessibility – in which case a simple, low cost biomarker test might be better suited? The point here is that there is a choice to make, a balance to reach between a sophisticated and a simple form of biomarker. Instead of striving for 'ideal' biomarkers that will solve altogether the biological, economic, social and ethical complexities around cancer, we argue that it is more constructive and fair to frame the scientific, political and social debates in terms of 'good enough' biomarkers. This means accepting that whatever our choices, there will be subsequent limitations to our biomarkers, depending on what we want to measure and why: the type of information we want to access and the purpose for which we are doing the test on a patient then and there. Indeed, framing cancer biomarkers as 'ideal' tools might give the impression that they can uncover the 'truth' about how cancer works and how it should be managed socially and economically. However, even our understanding of how normal cells work is incomplete. Human biology is complex, and all the research done on cancer so far has only revealed small parts of what is driving this disease. So the questions we should keep in mind are: for my purpose, what is a 'good enough' biomarker? When should I stop trying to make the biomarker more sophisticated without having a feeling of 'giving up' on patients? When does the biomarker help us make good enough and sensible medical, ethical and economic decisions; knowing that there always will be uncertainties and wherever we draw the line, there will always be people on the other side of the 'ragged edge' (Callahan, 1990), not receiving access to a particular treatment?

Framing cancer biomarkers in terms of 'good enough' tools might also help curb the 'culture of medicalisation' surrounding cancer. The attention to and promises of 'ideal' cancer biomarkers are a breeding ground for patients' hope and belief that "there are no inherent obstacles or pitfalls of science that could stop the realisation of revolutionary cures" (Brekke and Sirnes, 2011; p. 356); rather, policy-makers are criticised for refusing to invest the necessary resources into the different types of cancer. This optimism towards biomedical science is further illustrated by Callahan who talks about a 'mirage of health' (2003; p. 261): "Hope and reality have fused. Medical miracles are expected by those who will be patients, predicted by those seeking research funds, and profitably marketed by those who manufacture them. [...] The healthier we get, the healthier still we want to become. If we want to live to eighty, why not to one hundred? [...] The "mirage of health" – a perfection that never comes – is no longer taken to be a mirage, but solidly out there on the horizon." Introducing the notion of 'good enough' biomarkers might help temper these expectations in the face of cancer's high biological and social complexities, and help steer attention to questions such as: how should we, as a society, allocate limited resources in a fair way (see Chapters 4 and 5)? Or: what does it mean today to have cancer, and how should we care for these patients (see Chapter 7)? This is the role of 'good enough' biomarkers: to help reintroduce some human judgement – 'realism', 'reason', 'sensibility' and 'prudence' – (Callahan, 2003) into discussions of what we want from cancer research and care, when faced with our own certain mortality, and rich biological and social complexities.

5. Conclusion

The biology of cancer is extremely complex and uncertain, and the temptation equally high of seeing biomarkers as 'ideal' tools that will help us better understand this disease as well as guide better, safer, more sustainable and ethical medical decisions. However, we saw in this chapter that 'ideal' biomarkers that would solve all biological, social and economic complexities, and release us from having to address the tough ethical dilemmas of how to fairly allocate scarce health resources nationally and globally, are unattainable. Further, they create misleading hope among patients and shift social debates away from important questions around cancer research and care, such as what it means to be a cancer patient today, and how we should care for these patients.

Instead, we argue that talking in terms of 'good enough' biomarkers would help us acknowledge and address the complexities and uncertainties around cancer biology in a constructive way, and leave room for debating social and ethical questions in a context of personalised medicine. By encouraging discussions on what we as a society want out of cancer research and care, 'good enough' biomarkers are important contributions to the research and care in a context of personalised cancer medicine.

6. References

Alizadeh, A. A., Eisen, M. B., Davis, R. E., et al. (2000). Distinct types of diffuse large B-cell lymphoma identified by gene expression profiling. *Nature, 403*(6769), 503-511.

Blanchard, A. (2016). Mapping ethical and social aspects of cancer biomarkers. *New Biotechnology, 33*(6), 763-772.

Brekke, O. A., and Sirnes, T. (2011). Biosociality, biocitizenship and the new regime of hope and despair: interpreting "Portraits of Hope" and the "Mehmet Case". *New Genetics and Society, 30*(4), 347-374.

Callahan, D. (1990). *What Kind of Life: The Limits of Medical Progress.* Washington, D.C.: Georgetown University Press.

Callahan, D. (2003). *What Price Better Health? Hazards of the Research Imperative* (Vol. 9). Berkeley and Los Angeles, California: University of California Press.

Cancer Genome Atlas Research, Kandoth, C., Schultz, N., Cherniack, A. D. et al. (2013) Integrated genomic characterization of endometrial carcinoma. *Nature, 497*(7447), 67-73.

Cuzick, J., Dowsett, M., Pineda, S., et al. (2011). Prognostic value of a combined estrogen receptor, progesterone receptor, Ki-67, and human epidermal growth factor receptor 2 immunohistochemical score and comparison with the Genomic Health recurrence score in early breast cancer. *J Clin Oncol, 29*(32), 4273-4278.

Diamandis, E. P. (2012). The failure of protein cancer biomarkers to reach the clinic: why, and what can be done to address the problem? *BMC Med, 10,* 87.

Early Breast Cancer Trialists' Collaborative, Davies, C., Godwin, J., Gray, R., et al. (2011). Relevance of breast cancer hormone receptors and other factors to the efficacy of adjuvant tamoxifen: patient-level meta-analysis of randomised trials. *Lancet, 378*(9793), 771-784.

EC. (2013). *Commission staff working document on the use of 'omics' technologies in the development of personalised medicine.* Brussels: European Commission.

EC. (2015). *European Council conclusions on personalised medicine for patients.* Publications Office of the European Union, Luxembourg: European Council.

EC. (2016a). *Towards an International Consortium for Personalised Medicine (IC PerMed).* Brussels: European Commission.

EC. (2016b). *Personalised Medicine Conference 2016 Report.* Publications Office of the European Union, Luxembourg: Directorate General for Research and Innovation, European Union.

Fleck, L. M. (2012). Pharmacogenomics and personalised medicine: wicked problems, ragged edges and ethical precipices. *New Biotechnology, 29*(6), 757-768.

Fredriksen, S. (2006). Tragedy, utopia and medical progress. *Journal of Medical Ethics, 32*(8), 450-453.

Freidlin, B., McShane, L. M., Polley, M. Y., and Korn, E. L. (2012). Randomized phase II trial designs with biomarkers. *J Clin Oncol, 30*(26), 3304-3309.

Füzéry, A. K., Levin, J., Chan, M. M., and Chan, D. W. (2013). Translation of proteomic biomarkers into FDA approved cancer diagnostics: issues and challenges. *Clin Proteomics, 10*(1), 13.

Gerlinger, M., Rowan, A. J., Horswell, S., et al. (2012). Intratumour heterogeneity and branched evolution revealed by multiregion sequencing. *N Engl J Med, 366*(10), 883-892.

Golub, T. R., Slonim, D. K., Tamayo, P., et al. (1999). Molecular classification of cancer: class discovery and class prediction by gene expression monitoring. *Science, 286*(5439), 531-537.

Gutman, S., and Kessler, L. G. (2006). The US Food and Drug Administration perspective on cancer biomarker development. *Nat Rev Cancer, 6*(7), 565-571.

Hanahan, D., and Weinberg, R. A. (2011). Hallmarks of cancer: the next generation. *Cell, 144*(5), 646-674.

Helsedirektoratet. (2016). *Summary of the Norwegian strategy for personalised medicine in healthcare 2017-2021.* Oslo: Norwegian Directorate of Health (Helsedirektoratet).

HOD. (2016). *Prop. 1S HOD for Budsjettåret 2017.* Oslo, Norway: Helse- og Omsorgsdepartement [Ministry of Health and Care Services].

Jackson, D. B., and Sood, A. K. (2011). Personalised cancer medicine: Advances and socio-economic challenges. *Nature Reviews Clinical Oncology, 8*(12), 735-741.

Kern, S. E. (2012). Why your new cancer biomarker may never work: Recurrent patterns and remarkable diversity in biomarker failures. *Cancer Research, 72*(23), 6097-6101.

Krop, I. E., Kim, S. B., Gonzalez-Martin, A., et al. (2014). Trastuzumab emtansine versus treatment of physician's choice for pretreated HER2-positive advanced breast cancer (TH3RESA): a randomised, open-label, phase 3 trial. *Lancet Oncol, 15*(7), 689-699.

Li, W., Wang, R., Yan, Z., Bai, L., and Sun, Z. (2012). High accordance in prognosis prediction of colorectal cancer across independent datasets by multi-gene module expression profiles. *PLoS One, 7*(3), e33653.

Loi, S., Michiels, S., Baselga, J., et al. (2013). PIK3CA genotype and a PIK3CA mutation-related gene signature and response to everolimus and letrozole in estrogen receptor positive breast cancer. *PLoS One, 8*(1), e53292.

Majewski, I. J., and Bernards, R. (2011). Taming the dragon: genomic biomarkers to Microtubule-associated protein tau: a marker of paclitaxel sensitivity in breast cancer. *Proc Natl Acad Sci USA, 102*(23), 8315-8320.

Mordente, A., Meucci, E., Martorana, G. E., and Silvestrini, A. (2015). Cancer Biomarkers

Discovery and Validation: State of the Art, Problems and Future Perspectives. *Adv Exp Med Biol, 867*, 9-26.

Nakazawa, M., Lu, C., Chen, Y., et al. (2015). Serial blood-based analysis of AR-V7 in men with advanced prostate cancer. *Ann Oncol, 26*(9), 1859-1865.

Ni, X., Zhang, W., and Huang, R. S. (2013). Pharmacogenomics discovery and implementation in genome-wide association studies era. *Wiley Interdiscip Rev Syst Biol Med, 5*(1), 1-9.

NIH (2001). Biomarkers and surrogate endpoints: preferred definitions and conceptual framework. National Institute of Health Biomarkers Definition Working Group. *Clin Pharmacol Ther, 69*(3), 89-95.

Oshima, K., Naoi, Y., Kishi, K., et al. (2011). Gene expression signature of TP53 but not its mutation status predicts response to sequential paclitaxel and 5-FU/epirubicin/cyclophosphamide in human breast cancer. *Cancer Lett, 307*(2), 149-157.

Perou, C. M., Sorlie, T., Eisen, M. B., et al. (2000). Molecular portraits of human breast tumours. *Nature, 406*(6797), 747-752.

Polley, M. Y., Freidlin, B., Korn, E. L., et al. (2013). Statistical and practical considerations for clinical evaluation of predictive biomarkers. *J Natl Cancer Inst, 105*(22), 1677-1683.

Qi, Y., & Wang, W. (2016). Clinical significance of circulating tumor cells in squamous cell lung cancer patients. *Cancer Biomark*.

Ross, J. S., Slodkowska, E. A., Symmans, W. F., et al. (2009). The HER-2 receptor and breast cancer: ten years of targeted anti-HER-2 therapy and personalized medicine. *Oncologist, 14*(4), 320-368.

Rouzier, R., Rajan, R., Wagner, P., et al. (2005). Microtubule-associated protein tau: a marker of paclitaxel sensitivity in breast cancer. *Proc Natl Acad Sci U S A, 102*(23), 8315-8320.

Salvesen, H. B., Haldorsen, I. S., and Trovik, J. (2012). Markers for individualised therapy in endometrial carcinoma. *Lancet Oncol, 13*(8), e353-361.

Schechter, A. L., Stern, D. F., Vaidyanathan, L., et al. (1984). The neu oncogene: an erb-B-related gene encoding a 185,000-Mr tumour antigen. *Nature, 312*(5994), 513-516.

Schuster, C., Eikesdal, H. P., Puntervoll, H., et al. (2012). Clinical efficacy and safety of bevacizumab monotherapy in patients with metastatic melanoma: predictive importance of induced early hypertension. *PLoS One, 7*(6), e38364.

Slamon, D., Eiermann, W., Robert, N., et al. (2011). Adjuvant trastuzumab in HER2-positive breast cancer. *N Engl J Med, 365*(14), 1273-1283.

Swain, S. M., Baselga, J., Kim, S. B., et al. (2015). Pertuzumab, trastuzumab, and docetaxel in HER2-positive metastatic breast cancer. *N Engl J Med, 372*(8), 724-734.

TCGA Network (2012). Comprehensive molecular portraits of human breast tumours. *Nature, 490*(7418), 61-70.

Teutsch S.M., Bradley L.A., Palomaki G.E., et al (2009). The Evaluation of Genomic Applications in Practice and Prevention (EGAPP) Initiative: methods of the EGAPP Working Group. *Genet Med, 11*(1), 3-14.

van't Veer, L. J., Dai, H., van de Vijver, M. J., et al. (2002). Gene expression profiling predicts clinical outcome of breast cancer. *Nature, 415*(6871), 530- 536.

Vargas, A. J., and Harris, C. C. (2016). Biomarker development in the precision medicine era: lung cancer as a case study. *Nat Rev Cancer, 16*(8), 525-537.

Ventola, C. L. (2013). Role of pharmacogenomic biomarkers in predicting and improving drug response: part 1: the clinical significance of pharmacogenetic variants. *P T, 38*(9), 545-560.

Verma, S., Miles, D., Gianni, L., et al. (2012). Trastuzumab emtansine for HER2-positive advanced breast cancer. *N Engl J Med, 367*(19), 1783-1791.

2

ECONOMIC EVALUATIONS OF CANCER BIOMARKERS FOR TARGETED THERAPIES: PRACTICES, CHALLENGES, AND POLICY IMPLICATIONS

Mikyung Kelly Seo

1. Introduction

The health economic impact of cancer biomarkers for targeted therapies can be mainly divided into two aspects. First, it has clinical implications for patient outcomes by directing the right treatment to the right patient or by determining the treatment that would provide no or minimal health benefits to patients. Second, it has financial implications for patient care by avoiding any unnecessary costs that would be otherwise spent on. Given the high costs of cancer targeted therapies, the optimisation of treatment decisions would contribute to containing unnecessary costs without hurting patient outcomes, as patients unlikely to respond would not be exposed to toxicity or potential harms caused by cancer treatments.

With the increased understanding of genetics and molecular biology, the optimisation of treatment strategies is now possible based on the information provided by biomarkers prior to treatment (Nass and Moses, 2007, Trusheim et al., 2007). These advances have raised expectations concerning personalised medicine or precision medicine, which aims to

Anne Blanchard and Roger Strand (Eds.), *Cancer Biomarkers: Ethics, Economics and Society.* Bergen: Megaloceros Press, 2017. ISBN 978-82-91851-04-4 (paperback). https://doi.org/10.24994/2018/b.biomarkers © The Authors / Megaloceros Press.

provide the right treatment to the right patient. Biomarker-targeted drug development is most actively observed in oncology, leading to an increased number of potential cancer biomarkers tested in laboratories and clinical trials. Oncology treatments are currently at the frontline of this advancement showing promise in developing drugs based on an exact understanding of disease mechanisms. Table 1 presents some examples of cancer biomarkers for targeted therapies. These biomarkers can assist in making the optimal treatment decisions possible for the safe and effective use of corresponding drugs.

Cancer type	Biomarker	Example targeted therapies
Breast	HER2	Trastuzumab (Herceptin®), Lapatinib (Tyverb®), Pertuzumab (Perjeta®), Pabociclib (Ibrance®)
CRC	KRAS/RAS	Cetuximab (Eribitux®), Panitumumab (Vectibix®)
NSCLC	EGFR	Erotinib (Tarceva®), Gefitinib (Iressa®)
	ALK	Crizotinib (Xalkori®)
	PD-L1	Pembrolizumab(Keytruda®)
Melanoma	BRAF V600E	Vemurafenib (Zelboraf®), Dabrafenib (Tafinlar®)
	MEK	Trametinib(Mekinist®)

Table 1. Examples of cancer biomarkers for targeted therapies. Abbreviations: CRC, colorectal cancer; NSCLC, non-small-cell lung cancer.

A biomarker is defined as "a characteristic that is objectively measured and evaluated as an indicator of normal biological processes, pathogenic processes, or pharmacologic responses to a therapeutic intervention" (Colburn et al., 2001). Simply put, biomarkers have multiple applications in the care process. They can be used diagnostically, prognostically, or predictively, but the key part of cancer biomarkers for targeted therapies lies in their ability to inform clinicians whether a specific group of patients would respond or not prior to the provision of the corresponding therapies. In other words, they have great potential for optimising treatment decisions in clinical practice so that payers save unnecessary expenditures that provide no or minimal benefits to patients, while unresponsive patients can avoid unnecessary exposure to toxicity or potential harms. It is thus argued that precision medicine will eventually improve health outcomes for patients and help achieve resource allocation efficiency in health services. These predictive biomarkers are basically aimed toward stratifying patients into a subgroup of responders and non-responders to the corresponding therapies, as guided by the biomarker test results.

Despite such high expectations, there is widespread scepticism about the research and development (R&D) of biomarkers and personalised medicines in relation to the return of investments (ROI) for technology developers and the budget impact for healthcare payers. According to a Quintiles report (Quintiles, 2011), 56% of managed care executives feel that personalised medicines are likely to increase the costs of prescription drugs. Furthermore, the R&D investment in biomarkers becomes even more controversial when it comes to the success rate of published biomarkers entering clinical practice (Burke, 2016; Kern, 2012). A recent empirical study that investigated the number of predictive biomarkers licensed in Europe confirmed this scarcity as well (Malottki et al., 2014).

This chapter begins with an overview of existing economic evaluations conducted on cancer biomarkers focusing on methodological approaches. It then discusses methodological challenges and issues in conducting economic evaluations of cancer biomarkers without clear guidance on evidentiary standards and consensus on data requirements for economic evaluations. It concludes with some policy implications for regulatory and reimbursement bodies in order to ensure a timely integration of cancer biomarkers into clinical use.

2. Overview of existing economic evaluations on cancer biomarkers

Many biomarker tests struggle to gain market access and obtain appropriate coverage due to the lack of robust evidence on their health economic impact. Economic evaluations of diagnostics, such as biomarker tests, are far less frequently reported than for drugs. This small number of reports may relate to a paucity of biomarker tests routinely available in clinical practice. There are some systematic literature reviews (SLR) in relation to economic evaluations of biomarker testing. Wong et al. (2010) identified 34 economic evaluation studies on pharmacogenomics between the years of 1950 and 2009. This was a three-fold increase from the number of previous SLR study searched economic studies between 1950 and 2004 (11 studies identified) (Phillips and Van Bebber, 2004). It was then increased to 42 studies even though the time-span was reduced to 10 years (2000-2010)(Vegter et al., 2010). Moreover, a recent SLR identified 32 studies with only a 5-year timespan (Oosterhoff et al., 2016). This implies that a majority of economic evaluations on biomarker testing were done only recently, and most likely since 2004 (Wong et al., 2010). Yet, there are relatively few predictive biomarkers licensed despite the large body of literature and extensive research investments on potential biomarkers (Malottki et al., 2014).

Authors and search period	Studies inclu-ded	Study purpose	Primary finding	Quality assessment
Plothner et al. (2016): 2000-Nov 2015	27	To review the cost-effectiveness of PG guided drugs with and without prior genetic testing	PGx improves the cost-effectiveness of pharmacotherapy	QHES used and scored on average 85.81/100
Doble et al. (2015): Until Feb 2014	30	To review characteristics of companion diagnostics important for health economic modelling	The prevalence of the biomarker of interest, the patient population eligible for testing, the testing costs especially when prevalence is small, the sensitivity and specificity of a test, limited evidence, a test's threshold for positivity	QHES used and on average scored 73/100
Hatz et al. (2014): Until Feb 2013	84	To review the health economic evidence and the cost-effectiveness of IM	No clear evidence that IM using genetic testing is superior in cost-effectiveness	Not reported
Phillips et al. (2014): Until 2011	59	To review evidence on economic value of PM tests	Many studies reported that PM tests provide better health at a higher cost but few being cost-saving	Not reported
Phillips and Van Bebber (2004): Until 2004	11	To assess the value of PGx interventions	Test performance was a critical factor. Lack of discussion of the importance of clinical utility of testing, potential impact on societal health as a whole	Not reported

Table 2. Systematic reviews of economic evaluations on cancer biomarkers for targeted therapies. Abbreviations: IM, individualised medicine; PGx, pharmacogenetics/pharmacogenomic screening; PM, personalised medicine; QHES, quality of health economic studies.

Table 2 summarises a list of systematic reviews conducted on biomarkers for targeted therapies. All reviews identified a lack of quality in relation to data requirements for economic evaluation of biomarker tests, including clinical validity of biomarker testing and prevalence of the biomarker of interest. Many of the studies reported a positive impact of biomarker tests in improving the cost-effectiveness of targeted therapies, however, this did not necessarily mean that the inclusion of biomarker testing would guarantee the cost-effectiveness of the corresponding targeted therapies. For example, some of the targeted therapies still resulted in not being cost-effective even though the inclusion of biomarker testing helped to improve the cost-effectiveness of targeted therapies. In other words, the cost-effectiveness of cancer biomarkers seems to be largely driven by characteristics of targeted therapies rather than that of biomarkers. Cancer targeted therapies are often very expensive and their clinical effectiveness does not compensate such high costs. This is one of the major reasons why pharmaceutical industries are attracted to the development of biomarker technologies so that they may achieve cost-effectiveness of their drugs without reducing the price by targeting a subgroup of patients who are responsive to their drug of interest. Companion diagnostics (CDx) is an example of this successful integration into clinical use (Table 1). CDx are co-developed/tested in trials together with their corresponding therapies or are developed after a drug is made available on the market.

3. Methodological challenges and issues

While the basic principles for the economic evaluation of pharmaceutical drugs should be similarly applied to cancer biomarkers for targeted therapies, given the nature of the multiple applications of biomarker testing and their indirect impact on the clinical effectiveness and cost-effectiveness of corresponding therapies, test developers face some specific issues and methodological challenges. These challenges need to be addressed by decision makers with clarity on methodological approaches and evidentiary standards not only for regulatory approvals but also for reimbursement decisions in order to ensure a timely integration of biomarkers into clinical use. In this section, I will discuss methodological challenges and issues faced by test developers in the framework of economic evaluations.

In most countries, the procedure of health technology assessment (HTA) appraisal for diagnostics is separated from pharmaceutical drugs. However, few guidelines exist for the evaluation of precision medicine or co-dependent technologies. A general view seems to be that separate HTA guidelines for precision medicine is not needed. For example, the National Institute of Health and Care Excellence (NICE) in the UK has introduced a separate programme evaluating new diagnostic technologies (DAP, Diagnostic Assessment Programme) from that of drugs, but no separate guidelines exist for precision medicine or biomarkers for targeted therapies. NICE has so far seen no such needs but recommends application of the same HTA guidelines as for conventional pharmaceutical drugs to cancer biomarkers for targeted therapies. Until now, very few country-specific guidelines have been proposed for precision medicine. Australia is one of the very few countries to suggest a national framework for evaluating clinical evidence of co-dependent technologies (Merlin et al., 2013).

a. The viewpoint of the analysis

Economic evaluations are performed from a variety of perspectives such as that of the patient, the hospital, the health system, or the society. In most cases, economic evaluations are performed following country-specific guidelines for HTA with the viewpoint of third party payers such as national health services (NHS) in the UK or social health insurance systems in France and Germany. However, most evaluations on pharmacogenetic tests are done from an academic interest or hospital perspective, implying that cost-effectiveness studies of biomarkers are as of yet limited to academic interests rather than commercial purposes (Vegter et al., 2010). This observation is explained in part by less strict reimbursement processes for diagnostics compared to those for pharmaceutical drugs.

Defining the viewpoint of the analysis of new technologies is a starting point for economic evaluations. It determines the scope of relevant costs and health benefits to be assessed. Given the nature of the multiple applications and the indirect health impact of biomarkers on patient health, it could be desirable to take a holistic viewpoint rather than a third-party payer perspective. Its economic evaluation might then capture the full spectrum of health economic impact of biomarkers. This is important because cancer biomarkers for targeted therapies may realise a wider range of patient benefits in comparison to that of conventional pharmaceutical drugs. For example, it is of value to patients that they are informed of the most optimal treatments scientifically proven to be effective for them. Or, patients can be assured that their expected health benefits will be at a minimal or harmful level when they are excluded from the provision of the treatment. It is to patients' benefit that they do not need to be exposed to unnecessary harm or adverse events caused by treatment. It is, in the end, to the benefit of society that working aged populations can return to work quickly or avoid morbidity due to unnecessary exposure to adverse events of targeted therapies. A recent study (OHE, 2016) on the value of complementary diagnostics, including CDx, identified even more benefits, such as a reduction in uncertainty (additional value from knowing a technology is likely to work); the value of hope (willingness to accept greater risk); real option value (benefits from future technologies); insurance value (psychic value); and scientific spillover (knowledge spillover).

In sum, the value of cancer biomarkers needs to be viewed beyond direct benefits and costs incurred on health systems. A holistic viewpoint would be more appropriate in assessing the health economic impact of biomarkers in order to capture the full spectrum of health benefits and costs.

b. The choice of treatment alternatives (comparators)

Standard of care (SOC) is most widely used as a comparator in economic evaluations, according to the HTA guidelines in many countries. With regard to assessing the cost-effectiveness of biomarkers for targeted therapies, a 'treat-all strategy' is currently suggested as a comparator (Faulkner et al., 2012) and various economic evaluations on biomarker-guided targeted therapies have used the strategy of 'treat all patients with new technology' as a comparator arm (Fugel et al., 2016). A current practice seems to be that the value of cancer biomarkers for targeted therapies is expressed by that of corresponding therapies and often, it is not evaluated compared to SOC without biomarker testing.

According to Seo and Cairns (2016), the cost-effectiveness of cancer biomarkers is largely dependent on the choice of comparator strategy. If the strategy of 'test-treat' is compared with 'treat all patients with new treatment', it often shows that testing biomarkers prior to the administration of corresponding therapies is more cost-effective. However, it shows not being cost-effective when compared to 'treat all patients with existing therapies'. This implies that the cost-effectiveness of cancer biomarkers is largely driven by the characteristics of the corresponding therapies. Since the current practice of selecting a comparator strategy is a 'treat-all strategy' with new therapy without testing, biomarker-guided therapies are likely to be found cost-effective. 'Treating all patients with SOC without testing' needs to be a comparator to maintain consistency in methodological approaches across different types of health technologies.

c.   Measuring clinical effectiveness

The lack of clinical evidence in biomarker testing is one of the significant challenges to payers in making decisions on reimbursement and coverage. Payers expect to make reimbursement decisions based on robust clinical effectiveness evidence, however, test developers will not invest in generating such evidence unless they know that such expenditures would be recouped with reasonable levels of ROI. Reimbursement of diagnostics is often cost-based in many countries and HTA recommendations for diagnostics are typically not legally binding, while drugs must be commissioned following a positive recommendation. It often leads to low pricing of diagnostics or, even after a positive HTA decision, test developers are left to convince individual commissioners to purchase technologies, resulting in a delay of test implementation in clinical practice. The clinical value of biomarker tests can be assessed as shown in Table 3.

Analytic validity	Accuracy and reliability of a test in detecting the entity of interest (e.g. genotype/biomarker/analyte) in specimens, mostly in the laboratory setting.
Clinical validity	Accuracy of a test in detecting/predicting the phenotype or clinical disorder of interest. It refers to sensitivity and specificity of a test in diagnosing or predicting risk for a disorder.
Clinical utility	Usefulness to the patient care decision-making process by providing information in order to select right treatments or preventive measures for patients or family members.

Table 3: Biomarker tests' clinical value.

The lack of evidentiary standards in evaluating the clinical effectiveness of a biomarker test is one of the main limiting factors in relation to the integration of a biomarker test into clinical use. Clear evidence requirements should be formulated. No consensus currently exists on methodological approaches in measuring the clinical effectiveness of cancer biomarkers for targeted therapies. The standards for generating the clinical evidence of biomarker tests have not yet been clearly established. Furthermore, such evidence cannot be generated for free. Test developers would not invest in generating clinical evidence without clearly knowing that their investments will be recovered by a reasonable level of reimbursement or market access.

The following are examples of study designs to assess the clinical effectiveness of a biomarker test. Randomised clinical trials (RCTs) are regarded as the gold standard in generating clinical evidence. However, this type of study design is often not feasible or very expensive to conduct for test developers. Various approaches have thus been discussed over the past decades, including prospective RCTs and enrichment studies. I will discuss some of the advantages and disadvantages of different study designs.

First, prospective RCTs are the study design in which patients are randomly assigned to biomarker-guided arm and non-guided arm. Patients assigned to the guided arm will receive treatments as guided by biomarker testing results (i.e. test-positive patients receive new treatment and test-negative patients receive existing treatment). Meanwhile, patients in non-guided arm will be randomly treated by either the new treatment or the existing treatment without biomarker testing. This study design has advantages in its ability for demonstrating the difference of treatment effect of biomarker-guided strategy as compared to that of non-guided strategy. However, it requires a large number of patients and it is quite costly.

Second, an enrichment study is a trial design that recruit patients with positive biomarker results. Although all patients are tested, only biomarker positive patients are randomly assigned to either new treatment or existing treatment arms. In other words, after the initial testing, patients with biomarker negative results are excluded from the trial. Enrichment study design is useful for biomarkers (or mutations) with rarity, in which only a small number of patients exist. However, it cannot demonstrate the treatment effect in biomarker negative patients and thus is not definitely able to establish the predictive value of a biomarker. In addition, it may pose some ethical questions as to whether it is ethical for biomarker negative patients to be excluded from the trial, especially when the clinical effect of corresponding therapy has not been clearly established for test negative patients and no alternative therapies exist for them.

Third, a retrospective study uses archived sample tissues or specimens. This type of study is less costly and less time intensive, however, the specimens of interest may not be archived from previous studies or processing methods may not be reliable. This study design is useful when a prospective trial is not feasible.

Fourth, single arm trial is testing all patients first but only biomarker positive patients are enrolled and uniformly treated with a treatment. Biomarker negative patients are excluded from the trial. This type of study does not have a control arm and cannot provide data on test positive patient groups. In addition to these four types of studies, there are also longitudinal observation studies and modelling studies.

d. Measuring health outcomes

Quality adjusted life years (QALY) or life years saved is the preferred outcome measure in the health economic guidelines of many countries. QALYs are recommended by several HTA bodies, such as NICE in the UK and Norwegian Medicines Agency (NoMA) in Norway. The QALY is popular because it allows comparison of therapies across different disease areas and interventions. However, challenges emerge when it comes to the assessment of cancer biomarkers, because those QALYs and mortality are based on disease-specific or preference-based outcome measures that are derived from the average population. The current metrics in measuring the impact of new technologies on health status using population-based preferences do not permit to fully capture individual patient utility of the health outcomes of biomarker testing. Given the nature of precision medicine (or personalised medicine) guided by biomarker testing, how to valuate individual patient preferences would be the key in measuring health outcomes of cancer biomarkers, although it would give rise to public debates especially for public-funded payers. There is more of an emphasis on individual patient preferences in attributing values to biomarkers as compared to conventional drugs. For example, patients or patient family members could be informed of prognostic or diagnostic information related to their choice of therapeutic option. Or, they could be informed of a wider range of alternative therapies based on biomarkers. Also, with biomarker-based information, patient-centred medicine can be realised with patients having more of a sense of controlling their own therapeutic choices with better assistance in individualised information. To the contrary, it may also cause more anxiety to patients when a test predicts non-response to targeted therapies but no alternative therapies exist for them.

e. Resource use and costs

The costing methodology in economic evaluations depends on the perspective of analysis employed in economic evaluations and there should not be a fundamental difference in calculating the costs of cancer biomarkers from that of traditional pharmaceutical drugs. However, as explained earlier, the cost-effectiveness of cancer biomarkers needs to be assessed from a holistic viewpoint in order to capture the full spectrum of costs and health benefits relevant to cancer biomarkers for targeted therapies. Thus, not only direct costs but also indirect nonmedical costs should be considered in economic evaluations of cancer biomarkers. Direct costs of cancer biomarkers might include additional clinic visits due to testing, sample collections, laboratory testing, genetic counselling, costs of associated therapies, management costs for adverse events, and monitoring costs. Indirect costs might include productivity costs, time spent on seeking treatment, cost savings due to appropriate treatments (morbidity costs due to inappropriate treatment could be saved), or any other opportunity costs saved.

Another aspect of challenge in calculating the costs of cancer biomarker testing is in identifying the appropriate unit costs. There is no national reference cost list for laboratory tests, including genetic testing. The price is often set by negotiations between test developers and hospitals, or it is set freely by individual laboratories. Thus, it is likely to have large variations in the price of biomarker testing even within the same jurisdiction. For example, no national pricing tariff exists for tests in the UK.

Lastly, there might incur capital costs for the purchase of laboratory testing equipment or any other upfront infrastructure. If this is the case, it should be considered in evaluations as well. Biomarker tests would require economic evaluations to include a much wider range of cost items more frequently compared to that of traditional pharmaceutical drugs.

4. Discussion and policy implications

The issue of timely integration of biomarker tests into clinical practice should be discussed within the framework of HTA to ensure a reasonable level of reimbursement and coverage for test developers, because reimbursement decisions by payers are critical for the integration of biomarkers into clinical use. Despite most countries providing clear HTA guidelines for conventional pharmaceutical drugs, few guidelines are drawn for cancer biomarkers for targeted therapies. For example, NICE in the UK does not provide HTA guidelines for precision medicine (or co-dependent technologies) but it does suggest to evaluate following HTA guidelines of conventional pharmaceutical drugs. The only framework existent for assessing biomarker-guided therapies would be the one from Australia (Merlin et al., 2013), which has yet to be further developed. The absence of clear HTA guidelines tailored for precision medicine reflects the current reality of reimbursement bodies in many countries not keeping pace with the rapidly evolving medical technologies such as 'omics'-based therapies. This may potentially delay the improvement of patient outcomes and may cause harm to patients by delaying the timely introduction of new technologies into clinical practice.

Currently, there is no clear guidance on evidentiary requirements for measuring clinical outcomes of biomarker tests. Establishing such standards is critical for appropriate biomarker tests to be integrated in a timely fashion into clinical practice. The lack of evidentiary standards for clinical effectiveness of biomarker testing is also linked to reimbursement challenges when it comes to conducting economic evaluations of cancer biomarkers. In this respect, CDx are in the frontline of development being integrated into clinical routine because they are often co-developed and tested simultaneously with corresponding drugs in trials, generating the clinical evidence required in HTA appraisals. It is the best available example of successful clinical utility efforts in the field of biomarkers (Parkinson et al., 2014). For example, trastuzumab and HER2 testing has succeeded in obtaining concurrent regulatory approvals and ensuring reimbursement for both drug and test.

Reimbursement bodies make decisions based on robust evidence of clinical effectiveness and cost-effectiveness (i.e. whether such introduction of new technologies provide more cost-effective health benefits to patients in comparison with existing technologies). In other words, the lack of evidentiary standards for clinical utility influences payers' willingness to pay and cover the costs of new technologies such as biomarker tests for targeted therapies (Cohen and Felix, 2014; Hresko and Haga, 2012). However, technology developers would not invest in generating further evidence required for HTA without knowing that they can get a reasonable level of ROI. Usually, reimbursement bodies have encompassed new technologies especially with oncology targeted therapies and rewarded them with high levels of reimbursement and access to the market. However, this was not necessarily always the case for test developers unless biomarker tests were co-developed with corresponding drugs. This has led to a limited number of biomarker tests integrated into clinical practice.

We can then ask the question how we should deal with cancer biomarkers that are not even cost-effective at zero price. It is a question to be addressed given that such high costs of targeted therapies are prevalent in oncology. Drug makers aim to recouping their R&D expenditures on drug development and evidence generation for regulatory and reimbursement approvals by securing the highest possible price for their drugs, within the acceptable cost-effectiveness thresholds of respective countries. Therefore, it is plausible that CDx or biomarker tests would not be cost-effective even at zero cost since they are evaluated as part of targeted therapies in economic evaluations.

Given that the cost-effectiveness of cancer biomarkers is largely dependent on the characteristics of the corresponding therapies (Seo and Cairns, 2016), we can think of some scenarios in relation to the interaction between cancer biomarkers and targeted therapies in terms of cost-effectiveness and clinical effectiveness. The first scenario would be when the cost of corresponding therapy is too high. The corresponding therapy is already too expensive and thus it would be unlikely for a biomarker test to be cost-effective. The second scenario would be when the corresponding therapy increases survival but leads to higher maintenance costs for patients eligible for the treatment and biomarker test. The third scenario would be when the clinical effectiveness of corresponding therapies is not good enough. The fourth scenario would be when the corresponding therapy causes high cost adverse events at a later stage of treatment while increasing additional survival. The sixth scenario would be when the corresponding therapy needs to be administered in combination with high cost treatments.

Lastly, an early development of economic evaluation models would provide useful information to test developers especially by incorporating the value of information analysis, given that the technology development of cancer biomarkers requires high R&D investments, and often multiple candidate biomarkers are tested simultaneously in trials. It is important as part of a continuous effort in managing and directing future research efforts on an iterative basis over the entire span of technology development. This would ensure consistency in the decision-making process between clinical adoption and technology development efforts.

5. Conclusion

A timely integration of new biomarkers into clinical use will not become a reality unless there is a clear signal from the demand side (e.g. payers) that test developers' investment will be recouped with a reasonable level of ROI, which is often practiced through the HTA process of reimbursement and coverage in many countries. However, it requires for test developers to demonstrate robust evidence of health economic impact of biomarkers for targeted therapies. Therefore, in order to realise the timely integration, clear guidance and a consensus on methodological approaches and evidentiary standards need to be made and signalled to test developers especially for economic evaluations.

Biomarker characteristics captured in economic evaluations are often limited to the cost or the accuracy of tests. Often, only the costs of biomarker testing are reflected in current practice when assessing the cost-effectiveness of cancer biomarkers for targeted therapies. Clinical outcomes or clinical utilities of cancer biomarkers are often difficult to reflect in economic evaluations due to the limited data generated by clinical trials. RCTs are known as the gold standard in generating evidence of clinical effectiveness of treatments, however, such a design is often difficult or infeasible for biomarker tests. Therefore, alternative ways of generating evidence for the clinical utility of biomarker tests need to be established. The lack of evidentiary standards for the clinical evidence of biomarkers for targeted therapies may lead to a delay of biomarker tests entering clinical routine practice. It partially explains why the number of biomarkers available in clinical routine is so limited compared to the number of new biomarkers discovered and published in many journals.

The development of evidentiary standards and guidelines are critical to the timely integration of biomarker tests for targeted therapies into clinical routine. Without clear guidelines in generating evidentiary standards, it is difficult for test developers to invest in generating the evidence required by regulatory and reimbursement bodies. It is of public and private interest to make the technology affordable and available to patients in need. Biomarker tests can provide information that is beneficial in order to select the right treatment for the right patient and lead to the improvement of patient health outcomes and quality of life. Although some of the issues discussed in this chapter could be better addressed by other fields (for example, the clinical utility of biomarker testing), a consensus on methodological approaches and data requirements for economic evaluations of biomarkers is urgently needed in the field of health economics. Health economics is yet to reach a consensus on whether existing methods are sufficient to evaluate the health economic impact of cancer biomarkers for targeted therapies, or whether different methodological approaches might produce conflicting results on cost-effectiveness.

6. References

Berm, E. J., Looff, M., Wilffert, B., Boersma, C., Annemans, L., Vegter, S., Boven, J. F. and Postma, M. J. (2016). Economic Evaluations of Pharmacogenetic and Pharmacogenomic Screening Tests: A Systematic Review. Second Update of the Literature. *PLoS One, 11*(1), e0146262.

Burke, H. B. (2016). Predicting Clinical Outcomes Using Molecular Biomarkers. *Biomark Cancer, 8*: 89-99.

Cohen, J. P. and Felix, A. E. (2014). Personalized Medicine's Bottleneck: Diagnostic Test Evidence and Reimbursement. *J Pers Med, 4*(2), 163-175.

Colburn, W., V. G. DeGruttola, D. L. DeMets, G. J. Downing, D. F. Hoth, J. A. Oates, C. C. Peck, R. T. Schooley, B. A. Spilker and J. Woodcock (2001). Biomarkers and surrogate endpoints: Preferred definitions and conceptual framework. Biomarkers Definitions Working Group. *Clinical Pharmacol & Therapeutics*, 69: 89-95.

Doble, B., Tan, M., Harris, A. and Lorgelly, P. (2015). Modeling companion diagnostics in economic evaluations of targeted oncology therapies: systematic review and methodological checklist. *Expert Rev Mol Diagn, 15*(2), 235-254.

Faulkner, E., Annemans, L., Garrison, L., Helfand, M., Holtorf, A.-P., Hornberger, J., Hughes, D., Li, T., Malone, D. and Payne, K. (2012). Challenges in the development and reimbursement of personalized medicine—payer and manufacturer perspectives and implications for health economics and outcomes research: a report of the ISPOR Personalized Medicine Special Interest Group. *Value in Health, 15*(8), 1162-1171.

Fugel, H. J., Nuijten, M., Postma, M. and Redekop, K. (2016). Economic Evaluation in Stratified Medicine: Methodological Issues and Challenges. *Front Pharmacol, 7*, 113.

Hatz, M. H., Schremser, K. and Rogowski, W. H. (2014). Is individualized medicine more cost-effective? A systematic review. *Pharmacoeconomics, 32*(5), 443-455.

Hresko, A. and Haga, S. B. (2012). Insurance coverage policies for personalized medicine. *J Pers Med, 2*(4), 201-216.

Kern, S. E. (2012). Why your new cancer biomarker may never work: recurrent patterns and remarkable diversity in biomarker failures. *Cancer Res, 72*(23), 6097-6101.

Malottki, K., Biswas, M., Deeks, J. J., Riley, R. D., Craddock, C., Johnson, P. and Billingham, L. (2014). Stratified medicine in European Medicines Agency licensing: a systematic review of predictive biomarkers. *BMJ Open, 4*(1), e004188.

Merlin, T., Farah, C., Schubert, C., Mitchell, A., Hiller, J. E. and Ryan, P. (2013). Assessing personalized medicines in Australia: a national framework for reviewing codependent technologies. *Med Decis Making, 33*(3), 333-342.

Merlin, T., Farah, C., Schubert, C., Mitchell, A., Hiller, J. E. and Ryan, P. (2013). Assessing personalized medicines in Australia: a national framework for reviewing codependent technologies. *Medical Decision Making, 33*(3), 333-342.

Nass, S. J. and Moses, H. L. (2007). *Cancer biomarkers: the promises and challenges of improving detection and treatment.* Washington D.C.: National Academies Press.

OHE, O. o. H. E. (2016). *The value of knowing and knowing the value: Improving the Health Technology Asessment of Complementary Diagnostics.*

Oosterhoff, M., van der Maas, M. E. and Steuten, L. M. (2016). A Systematic Review of Health Economic Evaluations of Diagnostic Biomarkers. *Appl Health Econ Health Policy, 14*(1), 51-65.

Parkinson, D. R., McCormack, R. T., Keating, S. M., Gutman, S. I., Hamilton, S. R., Mansfield, E. A., Piper, M. A., Deverka, P., Frueh, F. W., Jessup, J. M., McShane, L. M., Tunis, S. R., Sigman, C. C., and Kelloff, G. J. (2014). Evidence of clinical utility: an unmet need in molecular diagnostics for patients with cancer. *Clin Cancer Res, 20*(6), 1428-1444.

Phillips, K. A., Sakowski, J. A., Trosman, J., Douglas, M. P., Liang, S. Y. and Neumann, P. (2014). The economic value of personalized medicine tests: what we know and what we need to know. *Genet Med, 16*(3), 251-257.

Phillips, K. A. and Van Bebber, S. L. (2004). A systematic review of cost-effectiveness analyses of pharmacogenomic interventions. *Pharmacogenomics, 5*(8), 1139-1149.

Plothner, M., Ribbentrop, D., Hartman, J. P. and Frank, M. (2016). Cost-Effectiveness of Pharmacogenomic and Pharmacogenetic Test-Guided Personalized Therapies: A Systematic Review of the Approved Active Substances for Personalized Medicine in Germany. *Adv Ther, 33*(9), 1461-1480.

Quintiles (2011). *Exploring the perceptions of value and collaborative relationships among biompharmaceutical stakeholders.*

Seo, M. K. and Cairns, J. (2016). *A systematic review of the cost-effectiveness of diagnostic biomarkers for metastatic colorectal cancer in the context of targeted therapies.* Methods for Evaluating Medical Tests and Biomarkers (MEMTAB) Symposium. Institute of Applied Health Research, University of Birmingham. Birmingham, UK: 66.

Trusheim, M. R., Berndt, E. R. and Douglas, F. L. (2007). Stratified medicine: strategic and economic implications of combining drugs and clinical biomarkers. *Nat Rev Drug Discov, 6*(4), 287-293.

Vegter, S., Jansen, E., Postma, M. J. and Boersma, C. (2010). Economic evaluations of pharmacogenetic and genomic screening programs: update of the literature. *Drug Development Research, 71*(8), 492-501.

Wong, W. B., Carlson, J. J., Thariani, R. and Veenstra, D. L. (2010). Cost effectiveness of pharmacogenomics: a critical and systematic review. *Pharmacoeconomics, 28*(11), 1001-1013.

3

ECONOMIC EVALUATION OF TARGETED THERAPIES FOR NON-SMALL CELL LUNG CANCER

John Cairns

1. Introduction

The aim of this chapter is to review the economic evaluation of biomarker-guided therapies in order to identify the challenges involved when assessing the cost-effectiveness of biomarker-guided therapy. This is achieved by a detailed examination of the economic evaluations of the treatment of non-small cell lung cancer (NSCLC). NSCLC is a good area for the study of the evaluation of cancer biomarkers because there are several biomarker-guided therapies that have been appraised in recent years. The conclusion reached is that all the challenges identified are also present in the appraisal of other therapies but that a number of these challenges are potentially greater for biomarker-guided therapies. There are other important economic questions about biomarkers and biomarker-guided therapies around the incentives for their development and introduction, in particular, what is the optimal level of activity and how is it best achieved. However, the focus of this chapter is solely on evaluation issues.

Lung cancer comprises non-small cell lung cancers (85–90%) and small cell lung cancers (approximately 10–15%). The non-small-cell cancers themselves are divided into squamous cell carcinomas (45%),

Anne Blanchard and Roger Strand (Eds.), *Cancer Biomarkers: Ethics, Economics and Society.* Bergen: Megaloceros Press, 2017. ISBN 978-82-91851-04-4 (paperback). https://doi.org/10.24994/2018/b.biomarkers © The Authors / Megaloceros Press.

adenocarinomas (45%) and large-cell carcinomas (10%). About 5% of patients with stage III or IV NSCLC have chromosomal alterations described as anaplastic lymphoma kinase (ALK) fusion genes. The treatments ceritinib and crizotinib selectively inhibit the ALK receptor tyrosine kinase. Mutations in the tyrosine kinase domain of the epidermal growth factor receptor (EGFR) have been correlated with improved responses to EGFR tyrosine-kinase inhibitors such as erlotinib, gefitinib, afatinib and osimertinib. These EGFR-TK inhibitors block the signal pathway involved in cell proliferation and by doing so slow the growth and spread of tumours. About 50% of Asians and 10% of non-Asians have activating EGFR mutations. Necitumumab is used for the treatment of EGFR-expressing squamous non-small cell lung cancer. Blocking EGFR necitumumab reduces the growth and spread of cancer. Finally, pembrolizumab is used to treat patients who over-express PD-L1. Blocking PD-L1 receptors pembrolizumab increases the ability of the immune system to kill cancer cells.

The starting point for the chapter is the observation that throughout much of the economy we are prepared to allow decisions regarding what to produce and how much to produce to be led by the market. Nevertheless, in most countries we are unwilling to leave decisions concerning the production and consumption of health care services entirely to the market. Economic evaluation is an important means of informing decision-making. The chapter is silent on how important economic aspects are vis-à-vis other considerations, in particular, the distribution of costs and benefits.

The different approaches that have been taken to assess cost-effectiveness are compared, particularly in terms of the structure of the model, extrapolation of survival, the valuation of health states, costs of the drugs and of biomarker testing. The main challenges to assessing cost-effectiveness are identified and how these can be addressed in the future as the focus of evaluation moves from broad groups of patients to smaller and smaller sub-groups is explored.

2. Economic evaluations of treatment for non-small cell lung cancer

The raw material for this review comes from a series of health technology appraisals conducted by the National Institute for Health and Care Excellence (NICE) in the past ten years. Thus, there is no attempt to conduct a systematic literature review of economic evaluations of biomarker-guided therapies. This restricted focus not only renders the task more manageable, but also takes advantage of the transparent and well-documented decision-making process followed by NICE. Extensive information is readily available on the economic evidence supplied by manufacturers, the independent critical review of this evidence and the considerations of the appraisal committee that were influential for the final recommendation. Furthermore, the existence of a NICE Reference Case (NICE, 2013a) and template for manufacturers' submissions of evidence (NICE, 2015a) facilitates the identification of common themes and any differences in approach to evaluation. Table 1 lists chronologically the technology appraisals of therapies for non-small cell lung cancer and highlights those with explicit involvement of biomarkers. It highlights the dramatic changes in the potential for treating those with non-small cell lung cancer. There are more therapies in the pipeline and thus the list is a snapshot of a dynamic process that is ongoing rather than complete. For example, NICE will shortly make recommendations for the use of pembrolizumab in untreated patients and nivolumab in previously treated non-squamous non-small cell lung cancer.

Year	Technology Assessment	Drug and indication
2007	124	pemetrexed for NSCLC
2008	162	erlotinib for NSCLC
2009	181	pemetrexed 1st line
2010	190	pemetrexed maintenance
	192	gefitinib 1st line locally advanced **EGFR-TK+**
2011	227	erlotinib maintenance monotherapy **EGFR-TK+**
2012	258	erlotinib (1st line) locally advanced/ metastatic **EGFR-TK+**
2013	296	crizotinib previously treated **ALK+**
2014	310	afatinib locally advanced/ metastatic **EGFR-TK+**
2015	347	nintedanib previously treated locally advanced/ metastatic
	374	gefitinib and erlotinib maintenance after prior chemo **EGFR-TK+**
2016	395	ceritinib previously treated **ALK+**
	402	pemetrexed maintenance
	403	ramucirumab previously treated locally advanced/ metastatic
	406	crizotinib untreated **ALK+**
	411	necitumumab untreated locally advanced/ metastatic **EGFR-expressing**
	416	osimertinib (1st line) locally advanced/ metastatic **EGFR-T790+**
	422	crizotinib previously treated **ALK+**
2017	428	pembrolizumab **PD-L1+** after chemotherapy

Table 1. NICE non-small cell lung cancer technology appraisals.

Economic evaluation takes different forms but the established approach for informing discussion concerning whether or not third party payers, such as the National Health Service in England, should provide a particular treatment, is to assess cost-effectiveness using the cost per additional quality-adjusted life-year (QALY) gained. The QALY combines two important aspects of health: expected survival and the expected nature of the survival (sometimes referred to as health-related quality of life). The quality adjustment associates scores with the different health states that a patient experiences. Conventionally, a scale where one represents the value of full health and zero the value associated with being dead is used. In the context of caring for patients with cancer, time spent progression-free is valued more highly than time spent with progressed disease, and the quality adjustment can also capture the impact of different treatments and of different adverse effects on the patients.

3. Modelling the effect of treatment

The foundation for any attempt to assess the cost-effectiveness of therapies to treat non-small cell lung cancer is a model to determine how much time patients are likely to spend in different health states given existing treatments and under a new treatment strategy. The most popular approach to date is to develop a very simple model distinguishing three health states: progression-free, progressed disease and dead. There have been only two elaborations on this basic approach. The evaluation of gefitinib (NICE, 2010) distinguished between progression-free patients whose condition was stable and those whose disease showed evidence of responding to treatment. Whereas, the evaluation of necitumumab (NICE, 2016b) distinguished three progression-free health states: induction therapy, maintenance therapy and off treatment. These minor differences are unlikely to have had much impact on the estimated cost-effectiveness since the average costs and effects assumed in the case of a single progression-free health state will recognise that some patients were responding and that some patients will be off treatment.

The models developed to estimate the cost-effectiveness of biomarker-guided treatments for non-small cell lung cancer have all been partitioned survival models. These models start by specifying the relationship between overall and progression-free survival and time (see Figure 1). These curves are used to estimate what proportion of the patient cohort will be in the different health states over time. The proportion with progressed disease is estimated using the difference between the overall survival and progression-free survival curves. Thus, overall survival is partitioned into progression-free survival and survival with progressed disease.

The models differ to some extent in terms of the length of the cycle and time horizon, with cycle lengths of one week, three weeks and one month being variously assumed. The time horizons modelled have ranged from five to 20 years. Generally, shorter time horizons will capture a higher proportion of the costs than of the benefits. Thus, it is argued that the time horizon should be long enough to capture any significant differences between treatments. A lifetime perspective is generally recommended, however, the longer the time horizon the greater is uncertainty regarding costs and effects, and so often, the time horizon is not set to accommodate the predicted survival of the entire cohort. While discounting does not reduce uncertainty it dampens the impact on the estimated cost-effectiveness.

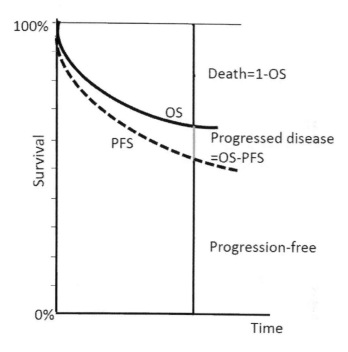

Figure 1. Partitioned survival model used in the appraisals of treatments for non-small cell lung cancer.

The modelling of survival has focused on estimating time spent progression-free and time spent with progressed disease because the costs of the two phases differ, in particular because treatment is generally discontinued on progression, and because health state utility values are higher for the progression-free state than for the progressed disease state.

Several challenges routinely arise when producing estimates of progression-free survival and overall survival for use in the modelling of costs and effects: extrapolation, adjusting for treatment switching and the need to make mixed or indirect treatment comparisons.

First, the limited duration of the relevant trials gives rise to the need to make projections regarding future events. In a typical trial patients are recruited at different points in time and followed up for different periods because analysis takes place at a point in time. Consequently, data are often censored, for example, some of the patients are still alive at the end of the follow-up period. Such censoring is important because it reduces the number of patients at risk (reducing the reliability of the estimated survival curve). The greatest effect is at the end of the curve where the maximum number of patients is censored. The Kaplan-Meier curve (see example in Chapter 4), a non-parametric estimator of the survival function, is widely reported in clinical trials and takes account of censored data. The Kaplan-Meier approach can only provide an estimate of the survival probability for the period of the observed follow-up. If economic evaluations were based only on the period of the trial follow-up they would be likely to produce misleadingly high costs per QALY gained (since they are likely to capture a higher proportion of the costs than of the benefits). Economic evaluations need to consider what happens to patients after the trial is completed. To achieve this, parametric survival functions are widely used to extrapolate a survival curve beyond the period of the trial. A wide range of standard functions have been used in the analyses of the treatments for non-small cell lung cancer: exponential, Weibull, Gamma, lognormal, Gompertz, log-logistic and generalised Gamma. It is important that the selected function provides a good fit for the observed data. Frequently more than one function can provide a satisfactory fit. In any case, it is not appropriate to base the selection of function solely on statistical criteria. It is necessary to consider the plausibility of the survival predictions that result from different functions and, where possible, to draw on external sources of data to justify a preference for one function over another. The selection of the parametric function with which to extrapolate the data is important because it can ultimately have a marked influence on the estimate of cost-effectiveness. For example, the estimated cost per QALY gained for osimertinib compared to pemetrexed plus cisplatin in the treatment of EGFR T790M mutation positive non-small cell lung cancer (NICE, 2016c) varies widely according to the survival model: lognormal (£31,289), log logistic (£43,299), exponential (£43,430), Weibull (£47,822), generalised Gamma (£145,984) and Gompertz (£1,052,785).

A second common problem arises because of treatment switching or crossover leading to biased estimates of the treatment effect (Latimer et al., 2014). This happens particularly in the control arm when patients receive the intervention drug following progression on the comparator drug. In such cases the estimates of progression free survival are not affected but treatment switching will generally lead to an underestimate of differences in overall survival. This creates problems for economic analysis because it requires accurate estimates of both progression-free survival and overall survival. Intention to treat analysis is likely to underestimate the treatment benefit. The submissions in the pembrolizumab and the three crizotinib appraisals made adjustments for treatment switching. The appraisal of crizotinib in untreated ALK positive patients (NICE, 2016a) is based on the PROFILE 1014 trial. Of the 171 patients randomised to pemetrexed plus cisplatin/carboplatin, 109 crossed over to crizotinib on disease progression. The hazard ratio for overall survival unadjusted for crossover was 0.821, compared to adjusted hazard ratios from 0.604 to 0.674 (depending on choice of method for adjusting for crossover). Two main approaches to adjusting the hazard ratio were considered in detail: the Rank Preserving Structural Failure Time Model and the use of a secondary baseline (or two-stage model). These two approaches make different assumptions, the former assumes a "constant treatment effect", that is, the treatment effect of crizotinib for those receiving crizotinib after progressing on chemotherapy is the same as for those patients receiving crizotinib at the outset. The latter approach assumes that there are "no unmeasured confounders" when estimating a treatment effect by comparing those who switch on progression with those that do not switch. In practice, it is often unclear which approach is superior but in this instance, they produced comparable results, and ultimately much more plausible estimates of incremental cost-effectiveness than using the unadjusted hazard ratio.

Third, there is often an absence of trials directly comparing the treatments of interest, which necessitates the use of indirect treatment comparisons. Indeed, it has been argued that even in the presence of trials directly comparing the two therapies of particular interest all relevant data should be considered since "[…] to ignore indirect evidence either makes the unwarranted claim that it is irrelevant, or breaks the established precept of systematic review that synthesis should embrace all available evidence" (Lu and Ades, 2004). About half of the evaluations have included indirect or mixed treatment comparisons. An indirect treatment comparison is where drugs A and B have both been compared to drug C and this common comparator is used to compare A and B indirectly. A mixed treatment comparison is where, in addition to such indirect comparisons, there are direct comparisons between the drugs of interest. For example, in the appraisal of necitumumab for untreated advance or metastatic EGFR-expressing squamous non-small cell lung cancer (NICE, 2016b) only one phase III trial was available. The SQUIRE trial compared necitumumab + gemcitabine + cisplatin with gemcitabine + cisplatin. An evidence network was constructed so that necitumumab could be compared with a wider range of treatments such as docetaxel + cisplatin and paclitaxel + carboplatin (see Figure 2).

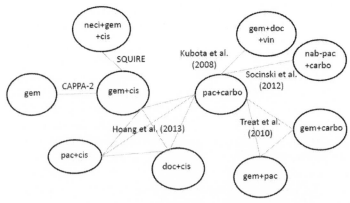

Figure 2. Evidence network for necitumumab. Based on Figure 23 of company evidence submission https://www.nice.org.uk/guidance/TA411/documents/committee-papers.

An important question arising with network meta-analyses is the extent to which the studies being compared are sufficiently similar to one another. In this example, only the SQUIRE trial was restricted to patients with squamous non-small cell lung cancer. Consequently, the evidence network compares the squamous sub-groups from these other trials. Across the different studies there are differences in the length of follow-up and in the proportion of patients with poorer performance status. Also in the necitumumab example, it is not possible to check that the direct and indirect comparisons are producing consistent estimates of the treatment effect since only the SQUIRE trial had a necitumumab arm.

All of these challenges are also present when appraising non-biomarker-guided therapies. The methods developed to address issues around extrapolation, treatment switching and absence of head-to-head trials clearly work better with more data rather than less and thus the appraisal of biomarker-guided therapies is more vulnerable to these challenges than is the appraisal of standard therapies.

4. Valuing health states

In all of these appraisals cost-effectiveness is measured by the cost per quality-adjusted life-year (QALY) gained. In order to estimate the QALYs gained by different treatments, health state utility values are used to weight the time spent in different health states. These values are conventionally expressed on a scale with one being the value attached to perfect health and zero to death. Thus, the better the health state a patient experiences the greater the number of QALYs generated.

Three different approaches have been used to value non-small cell lung cancer health states. The most widely used method involved the collection of EQ-5D data from patients in the trials of crizotinib, afatinib, osimertinib, necitumumab and pembrolizumab. The EQ-5D comprises single item questions about mobility, self-care, usual activities, pain/discomfort and anxiety/depression. These patient descriptions of their health state are then valued using a tariff or value set determined by the preferences of the general population. The preferences of the general population are used rather than those of patients because in a publicly-funded system taxpayers pay for the provision of health services and because use of a common set of values will facilitate consistent decision-making. An example of this approach is the appraisal of pembrolizumab (NICE, 2017) which used EQ-5D data collected during the KEYNOTE-010 trial when the patients were on treatment, at treatment discontinuation and 30 days later. These responses were valued using the UK tariff, and mean scores were calculated pre-progression and post-progression distinguishing between those ≥ 30 days and < 30 days from death.

The second approach, used in the appraisal of erlotinib and gefitinib, involves the direct valuation of cancer specific health states. Three of the appraisals (TA192, TA258 and TA374) took values from a study by Nafees et al. (2008) which had obtained values from 100 members of the UK general population for seventeen health states: eight stable states (seven with side effects); eight responding states (seven with side effects); and progressive disease, using standard gambles. With standard gambles, the risk of immediate death is varied until individuals are indifferent between the gamble and the certainty of experiencing the health state. In NICE's hierarchy of preferred approaches to health state valuation this is the least preferred approach, primarily because it reduces the comparability of evaluations.

Mapping algorithms are a third means of obtaining health state utility values, sometimes used when such data have not been directly collected. The appraisal of erlotinib monotherapy (TA227) used FACT-L data collected in the SATURN trial to estimate health state values. This was done by combining an algorithm developed from a dataset containing Visual Analogue Scale (VAS) scores provided by the general public for different FACT-L health states, and another algorithm to map thee VAS scores to the UK EQ-5D value set. The appraisal of ceritinib (TA395) used a mapping algorithm developed from EQ-5D and QLQ-C30 data collected from 154 multiple myeloma patients. The QLQ-C30 is a widely used cancer-specific questionnaire about the patient's experience during the past week, covering items such as nausea and vomiting, and physical and emotional functioning. This algorithm was then used to convert QLQ-C30 data collected in the ASCEND-2 trial into an EQ-5D equivalent. Mapping is potentially attractive in that it starts from condition-specific data but ends up with familiar and potentially comparable EQ-5D values. Comparability is clearly important for bodies making decisions across a wide range of clinical areas. For this reason mapping is preferred to directly valued condition-specific health states. This advantage comes at the cost of increased uncertainty because of uncertainty regarding the algorithm used to map from one to another. An alternative approach to mapping from cancer specific scales is to re-weight these cancer-specific responses using individuals' preferences over different aspects of health to produce condition-specific (in this case cancer) QALYs, for example, the EORTC-8D (Rowen et al. 2011). To date this approach has not been used in the appraisal of non-small cell lung cancer treatments.

Table 2 reports the range of values observed in the set of appraisals for the pre-progression and post-progression health states (30 days or more from death). There is a tendency for the values assigned to the post-progression health state to be higher when using EQ-5D data reported by patients in the trials. Although the values imply greater variability arising when the EQ-5D is collected directly from the patients in the trials, this is misleading because the directly valued and mapped values are based on many fewer studies. While this picture of differing health state values is not particular to biomarker-guided therapies, it highlights the point that use of an agreed set of values could improve comparability of appraisals. However, where there is robust evidence of better patient experience on-treatment with particular drugs, this needs to be reflected in the appraisal.

	Pre-progression	Post-progression
EQ-5D reported by patients in trials	0.653 – 0.815	0.517 – 0.678
Directly valued health state descriptions	0.653 – 0.673	0.473
EQ-5D mapped from cancer-specific measures	0.713 – 0.749	0.46 – 0.47

Table 2. Health State Utility Values

5. Costs of targeted therapies for non-small cell cancer

The most significant challenges with respect to estimating costs concern identifying the quantity of each drug which would be used (e.g. what proportion of patients receive the recommended treatment, extent of vial sharing/wastage, and duration of treatment). Often treatment is continued until disease progression and so there is no standard course of treatment. In the appraisal of osimertinib (NICE, 2016c) it was noted that sometimes patients continue to receive osimertinib beyond progression, so long as they are perceived to be receiving clinical benefit. In this appraisal the importance of treatment duration was such that it was recognised as a key area of interest for future data collection and formed part of a Managed Access Agreement on entry to the new Cancer Drugs Fund.

Depending on the drug adoption/reimbursement system the actual unit cost paid may not be readily available. For example, in England, afatinib, ceritinib, crizotinib, erlotinib, nintedanib, osimertinib and pembrolizumab all have Patient Access Schemes which involve a confidential discount on the list price. Such confidential discounts are attractive to manufacturers because they allow the official list price to remain unchanged. The Patient Access Scheme for gefitinib involves a fixed cost of treatment per patient (except where duration of treatment is <3 months and is free).

While, at first sight, identifying the costs of testing mutation status might appear to be straightforward, in practice, this has not proved to be wholly so. The first issue to consider is whether the costs of testing should be included. They have been included in the three crizotinib appraisals but there could be a question regarding at what point a particular test becomes part of routine clinical practice and less associated with a specific treatment. The committee accepted the argument that the cost of ALK testing is not relevant in the case of ceritinib because the relevant patient population will already have had crizotinib, and will thus have already been tested (NICE, 2016a).

In the crizotinib appraisals, it was assumed that all NSCLC patients would be tested, although most of the ALK positives are expected to be in the adenocarcinoma group. Testing was assumed to involve immunohistochemistry (IHC) with confirmation of equivocal results (IHC 1+ or 2+) using a fluorescence in-situ hybridisation (FISH) test. The cost of finding an ALK positive case will thus depend on, among other factors, the prevalence of ALK positivity and the proportion of equivocal IHC tests. It has generally been assumed that the prevalence of ALK positives is 3.8 per cent, implying that on average 29 patients need to be tested in order to identify an ALK positive case (NICE, 2016b). The estimated cost of ALK testing was £630 in TA296 (NICE, 2013b), between £2,380 (manufacturer) and £4,500 (evidence review group) in TA406 (NICE, 2016b). In the most recent crizotinib appraisal, neither the appraisal committee, nor the evidence review group, challenged the manufacturer's estimated cost of £1,638 per ALK-positive case identified. Possibly recognising that there were much more important uncertainties regarding the modelling of survival and duration of treatment, particularly, as in the crizotinib example, the cost of testing compared to the cost of the treatment itself is relatively low.

6. Economic evaluation with or without biomarkers

This chapter has highlighted some of the challenges to be faced when assessing the cost-effectiveness of biomarker-guided therapies for non-small cell lung cancer. Particular emphasis has been given to the challenges of extrapolating progression-free and overall survival, of identifying treatment effects, of valuing health states and of estimating costs over the long-term. However, it is important to note that all of these challenges to establishing cost-effectiveness noted above also feature prominently in evaluations of other treatments for non-small cell lung cancer. At first sight, there are no substantial differences.

However, there are a number of features that suggest that, while there are no specific differences in terms of assessing cost-effectiveness, economic evaluations of biomarker-guided therapies are likely to prove more difficult. Whether or not biomarker-guided therapies are systematically more costly, there are good grounds to anticipate that they would be. First, the number of patients for whom a therapy is potentially relevant may be smaller and thus the quantity that it is possible to sell may be less and higher per unit prices might be a strategy for recovering the cost of drug development. Second, targeted therapies might be regarded as offering eligible patients greater benefit and as reducing the number of patients who receive the adverse events associated with treatment with any compensating health improvement. Both these features might be viewed as warranting a higher price.

The stratification of treatment attendant on increasing use of biomarkers has other consequences. Trials of biomarker-guided therapies will have smaller numbers of patients, with increased problems with providing robust estimates of clinical effectiveness and increased uncertainty around estimates of cost-effectiveness. The way in which the relevant patient population is reduced by stratification can be illustrated with data for England, where annually about 17,000 patients present with locally advanced or metastatic non-small cell lung cancer. The number of patients in England each year whose cancer has the T790M mutation and whose cancer has progressed after receiving a first line EGFR TK inhibitor is estimated to be about 400. About 300 ALK positive patients each year are eligible to receive ceritinib, and the estimate for afatinib is about 450 patients per year, whereas roughly 2,000 patients per year whose tumours express PD-L1 are potentially eligible for treatment with pembrolizumab.

Some of the challenges encountered when identifying the impact of the introduction of biomarkers to guide therapy can be illustrated with the example of erlotinib. In TA162 (NICE, 2008) erlotinib was recommended as an alternative to docetaxel as a second line treatment for advanced/metastatic non-small cell lung cancer only if the treatment costs were the same. It was not recommended for second line use if docetaxel was either contraindicated or could not be tolerated. The Incremental Cost Effectiveness Ratio (ICER) versus Best Supportive Care (BSC) was £78,300. Also, it was not recommended for third line after docetaxel (ICER versus BSC £54,200). Erlotinib subsequently received European Medicines Agency approval for use as maintenance monotherapy in patients with stable disease after four cycles of platinum-based first line chemotherapy. However, this usage was not recommended by NICE (NICE, 2011), since the appraisal committee believed that the estimated ICERs for squamous and non-squamous non-small cell lung cancer versus BSC would be greater than £44,800 and £68,100 (and "considerably above" £50,000 for the whole stable population). Erlotinib was recommended as a first line treatment in patients with EGFR-TK positive cancer in June 2012 (NICE, 2012). This judgement was based on an assumption of equal clinical benefit between erlotinib and gefitiinib and the price discount on offer for erlotinib. Then in December 2015, erlotinib was not recommended as a second line treatment for EGFR-TK negative cancers in patients for whom docetaxel is suitable (NICE, 2015b). The evidence suggested that the costs were higher and the benefits were lower for erlotinib compared to docetaxel. A major contributor to this was the 90 per cent reduction in the price of docetaxel following the introduction of generic docetaxel. Erlotinib was also not recommended in those patients for whom docetaxel was unsuitable (the ICER versus BSC was likely to be over £50,000). However, erlotinib was recommended as an option in EGFR-TK positive cancer that had progressed in people who had received non-targeted chemotherapy and in specific circumstances for patients with unknown EGFR-TK mutation status.

In summary, docetaxel was initially approved for second line use and subsequently this was restricted to the treatment of EGFR-TK positive cancers (and some with unknown EGFR-TK positive status), and when erlotinib was approved for first line use this was restricted to EGFR-TK positive cancers. In trying to understand the impact of the introduction of a biomarker it would be instructive to compare the estimated QALY gains for all patients, and for patients with EGFR-TK positive and EGFR-TK negative cancers. Unfortunately, the estimates from TA162 and TA374 are essentially not comparable because of the use of different sources of data and the use of different estimation methods. For example, those receiving docetaxel second line are predicted to receive 0.2362 QALYs in the TA162 (all patient) appraisal compared with 0.5939 QALYs predicted for EGFR-TK negative patients in the TA374 appraisal. A clearer picture of the consequences for health outcomes of using EGFR-TK mutation status to guide erlotinib use would require use of a common set of methods to a common evidence network.

The increasing number of treatments, potentially available to the different strata of the overall patient population, is reflected in an increasing number of adoption/reimbursement decisions to be made, which makes consistent decision making more challenging. One aspect of this is the increasing number of drugs leading to an increased number of treatment sequences to be evaluated. Specific treatment sequences will become relevant to smaller and smaller groups of patients, further increasing the challenges of providing robust data on the effectiveness of different treatments. These challenges are beginning to be addressed with new clinical trial designs, such as umbrella studies of single tumour types, which compare the use of different combinations of biomarkers and drugs, and basket studies which focus on fewer marker-drug combinations but across a range of tumour types (Biankin et al., 2015).

Maintaining consistency in decision making over a sequence of new medicines and a series of decisions as the patient group changes, and similarly as the position in the clinical pathway changes, would be greatly facilitated if there were closer agreement over the methods to be used and if more of the parameter values were common across models. The desire to ensure consistency across decisions led NICE to specify a *Reference Case* "that specifies the methods considered by the Institute to be appropriate for the Appraisal Committee's purpose and consistent with an NHS objective of maximising health gain from limited resources" (NICE 2013a, p. 31). Nevertheless, within a specific clinical area, such as non-small cell lung cancer, the appraisals feature a variety of approaches and differing assumptions reducing comparability across studies (albeit while largely remaining within the *Reference Case*). An alternative approach that could directly address issues of consistency would be greater use of multiple technology appraisals, where all of the relevant drugs are considered at the same time (with the evidence on clinical and cost effectiveness produced by an independent assessment group) rather than sequentially with individual manufacturers making the case for their product. A disadvantage of this alternative is that new medicines would take a longer time to become part of routine clinical practice. Moreover, the drugs which obtained earlier regulatory approval would experience the greatest delay, weakening rather than strengthening the incentives to develop innovative medicines.

7. Conclusion

The challenges present when assessing the cost-effectiveness of biomarker-guided therapy are just the same as those in the absence of biomarkers. However, on occasion the challenges may be greater, primarily because of the tendency for treatment to become more stratified. This can have an impact on economic evaluation: the estimates of clinical effectiveness which are an important part of establishing cost-effectiveness may tend to become less precise, a process reinforced by the increasing fragmentation of care with increasing matching of biomarkers to therapeutic options and the increase in the number of different treatment sequences. The challenges of ensuring consistent decision-making across a series of appraisals, which are already present, will be increased rather than lessened.

8. References

Biankin, A. V., Piantadorsi, S., and Hollingsworth, S. J. (2015). Patient-centric trials for therapeutic development in precision oncology. *Nature, 526,* 361-70.

Latimer, N. R. et al. (2014). Adjusting survival time estimates to account for treatment switching in randomized controlled trials – an economic evaluation context: methods, limitations and recommendations. *Medical Decision Making, 34,* 387-402.

Lu, G. and Ades, A. E. (2004). Combination of direct and indirect evidence in mixed treatment comparisons. *Statistics in Medicine, 23,* 3105-3124.

Nafees, B., Stafford, M., Gavriel, S., Bhalla, S., and Watkins, J. (2008). Health state utilities for non small cell lung cancer. *Health and Quality of Life Outcomes, 6,* 84.

NICE (2008). Erlotinib for the treatment of non-small-cell lung cancer (TA162). https://www.nice.org.uk/guidance/ta162

NICE (2010). Gefitinib for the first-line treatment of locally advanced or metastatic non-small-cell lung cancer (TA192). https://www.nice.org.uk/guidance/ta192

NICE (2011). Erlotinib monotherapy for maintenance treatment of non-small-cell lung cancer (TA227). https://www.nice.org.uk/guidance/ta227

NICE (2012). Erlotinib for the first-line treatment of locally advanced or metastatic EGFR-TK mutation-positive non-small-cell lung cancer (TA258). https://www.nice.org.uk/guidance/ta258

NICE (2013a). Guide to the methods of technology appraisal 2013. https://www.nice.org.uk/process/pmg9/resources/guide-to-the-methods-of-technology-appraisal-2013-pdf-2007975843781

NICE (2013b). Crizotinib for previously treated non-small-cell lung cancer associated with an anaplastic lymphoma kinase fusion gene (TA296). https://www.nice.org.uk/guidance/ta296

NICE (2015a). Single Technology Appraisal: User Guide for Company Evidence Submission Template. https://www.nice.org.uk/process/pmg24/chapter/instructions-for-companies

NICE (2015b). Erlotinib and gefifitinib for treating non-small-cell lung cancer that has progressed after prior chemotherapy (TA374). https://www.nice.org.uk/guidance/ta374

NICE (2016a). Ceritinib for previously treated anaplastic lymphoma kinase positive non-small-cell lung cancer (TA395). https://www.nice.org.uk/guidance/ta395

NICE (2016b). Crizotinib for untreated anaplastic lymphoma kinase-positive advanced non-small-cell lung cancer (TA406). https://www.nice.org.uk/guidance/ta406

NICE (2016c). Necitumumab for untreated advanced or metastatic squamous non-small-cell lung cancer (TA411). https://www.nice.org.uk/guidance/ta411

NICE (2016d). Osimertinib for treating locally advanced or metastatic EGFR T790M mutation-positive non-small-cell lung cancer (TA416). https://www.nice.org.uk/guidance/ta416

NICE (2016e). Crizotinib for previously treated anaplastic lymphoma kinase-positive advanced non-small-cell lung cancer (TA422). https://www.nice.org.uk/guidance/ta422

NICE (2017). Pembrolizumab for treating PDL1-positive non-small-cell lung cancer after chemotherapy (TA428). https://www.nice.org.uk/guidance/ta428

Rowen, D., Brazier, J., Young, T., Gaugris, S., Craig, B. M., King, M. T., and Velikova, G. (2011). Deriving a preference-based measure for cancer using the EORTC QLQ-C30. *Value in Health, 14*, 721-31.

4

HOW CAN BIOMARKERS INFLUENCE PRIORITY SETTING FOR CANCER DRUGS?

Eirik Tranvåg and Ole Frithjof Norheim

1. Introduction

The ethics of priority setting in health care addresses the normative foundations for allocating resources in health. The level of scarcity may be relative, but even in high-income countries the need for priority setting is evident. Despite increasing budgets there will be conflicting interests that must be resolved through priority setting. A growing population of the elderly, new technologies and treatments, rising costs and increasing expectations from the public are drivers that create a health gap – a gap between what is medically possible and what is sustainable for a health care system.

Priority setting can be defined as the "ranking of patients or health services in order of importance" (Norheim 2016). Such a ranking, combined with resource constraints, may restrict beneficial treatment to patients and can potentially have substantial consequences. The reasons and arguments behind these must therefore be good and fair. But what is a good and fair decision? Is a good decision always fair? Is a fair decision always good?

Cancer research and treatment is at the frontier of what is medically

Anne Blanchard and Roger Strand (Eds.), *Cancer Biomarkers: Ethics, Economics and Society.* Bergen: Megaloceros Press, 2017. ISBN 978-82-91851-04-4 (paperback). https://doi.org/10.24994/2018/b.biomarkers © The Authors / Megaloceros Press.

possible. In the last years, innovations in cancer research have pushed and challenged what is sustainable for health care systems. Costly medicines with potentially large benefits for an unidentified subgroup of patients challenges the methods and toolbox we have for priority setting.

Biomarkers can help tailor cancer treatment. They can help us direct correct treatments to the correct patient at the correct time, and thereby increase the probability of success and reduce side effects and unnecessary treatments. We believe biomarkers also have the potential to improve priority setting for cancer treatment, and in this book chapter we will try to explain how this may happen.

First, we present a normative framework for commonly accepted principles and criteria for health care priority setting. Then we give a brief introduction to recent developments and discussions of priority setting in Norway. Then we discuss how biomarkers can potentially influence the three accepted criteria for priority setting in Norway, and in the last section we use the recent approval of a the PD-L1 inhibitor pembrolizumab for treatment of advanced non-small cell lung cancer (NSCLC) in Norway as a case study to illustrate both advantages and challenges of biomarkers in the priority setting process. We acknowledge that there are other and more established biomarkers in clinical use. Still, we chose this case as it is new, relevant and is central in the present debate on priority setting, resource use, and new and expensive cancer treatments.

2. Background theory

In this section we will give a very brief introduction to central concepts in normative theory relevant for the understanding of priority setting, and we will discuss important principles and criteria.[1] This will serve as background knowledge for the rest of the chapter.

a. Principles for priority setting

Consequentialism is the normative ethical theory that has been best developed for use in priority setting. In this view, what is considered a moral act depends on the consequence of that act. This contrasts with the other main approach in normative ethics: deontology, which emphasizes duties or rules (this is of course an oversimplification, but is sufficient in

---

[1] There may be reasonable disagreement over which criteria are relevant, how they should be interpreted, and how they should be weighted. It is easier to accept and settle for a decision if everyone can agree that the process leading to the decision is legitimate Daniels, N. and J. E. Sabin (2008). *Setting limits fairly: learning to share resources for health*, Oxford University Press.. This is important, but in this chapter we will not discuss the relation between biomarkers and a legitimate process.

our context). In the ethics of priority setting there has emerged a relative degree of consensus over which combinations of ethical considerations are relevant (these include a combination of consequentialist reasons and deontological constraints), and based on these, a set of principles have been developed. A principle can be defined as a rule or view governing one's behaviour (Oxford Dictionary 2017), which in the context of priority setting can be seen as a rule that specifies how interventions (or patients) should be ranked.

One of the core principles of priority setting is health maximization (Williams 1988, Ord 2012). According to this principle, priority should be given to interventions that maximize health benefit. This principle emphasizes the consequence (health benefit) of an action (prioritization), hence it is a consequentialist principle. The argument for this principle is intuitively easy to accept: given a limited amount of resources, an intervention that provides more health is preferred to an intervention that provides less health. Often this principle is operationalized through variants of the cost-effectiveness criterion. On its own, most consider the principle of health maximization insufficient as a base for priority setting. It does not consider whether the *distribution* of health benefits is fair.

Fair distribution is another core principle for priority setting (Brock and Wikler 2006). In this lies the view that it is not irrelevant to whom the health benefits are distributed, meaning that maximizing health is not the only morally relevant principle. Extra priority should be given to interventions benefiting those that are worse off. In health, those worse off are typically identified through criteria like severity or need. Arguments for fair allocation can be justified by the ideal of equality: resources should be allocated so that it reduces inequality in health outcomes (Temkin 1993, Arneson 2013). Another way of supporting this principle is through prioritarianism (Parfit 1997).

In addition, principles of impartiality and formal equality are fundamental: priority decisions being made must be unprejudiced and unbiased, and people who are equal in all relevant aspects should be treated equally.

b. *Criteria for priority setting*

A myriad of potential criteria for priority setting exist, and not all build on normative principles. Some are widely accepted as good and fair, others are seen as morally irrelevant and discriminatory, while some are disputed and contested. Despite this, criteria from all three groups are widely in use. For an overview, see Box 1.

Ethical aspects of priority setting

Key principles

1. Priority setting should aim at both fair distribution and health maximization

2. Priority setting should be impartial, unprejudiced, and unbiased

3. The formal principle of equal treatment
   - People who are equal in all relevant respects should be treated equally (horizontal equity), and
   - People who are unequal in the relevant respects should be treated unequally (vertical equity)

Relevant criteria for priority setting
   - Magnitude of health effect
   - Alternative cost
   - Health without the service in question (severity of disease)

Irrelevant criteria
   - Gender
   - Race
   - Ethnicity
   - Religion
   - Sexual orientation
   - Social status

Contested criteria
   - Age
   - Responsibility for own health
   - Area of living
   - Personal income

Box 1. Ethical aspects of priority setting

A health benefit or health effect criterion (the magnitude of health effect) is widely accepted and is motivated both by the health maximization and the fair distribution principle. Health benefit is often quantified using some summary measure of health, like quality adjusted life years (QALYs) gained or disability adjusted life years (DALYs) averted (Gold et al. 2002). They both incorporate measures of mortality and morbidity, making comparisons between different diseases and health states possible.

Another accepted criterion is cost, resource use or opportunity cost. The cost criterion is sometimes criticized for being non-medical and therefore irrelevant (Williams 1992), but it is in fact crucial for operationalization of the health maximization principle. Calculations of cost-effectiveness are central to priority setting. A cost-effectiveness ratio is calculated by dividing an interventions' cost by its effect (usually measured in QALYs). The output of the calculation is not, unlike what many claim, the value of a life. It is how much extra in terms of resources are needed to gain one additional unit of health. This can literally be seen as the lowest common denominator for comparing health outcomes: if intervention A has a cost-effectiveness ratio that is twice as high as intervention B, it requires twice as much resource to gain one quality adjusted life year. According to the health maximization principle, intervention B should be given priority. The opportunity cost of selecting intervention A is twice the amount of health one could have gained from intervention B.

A third widely accepted criterion, both among clinicians and in the public, is severity of disease, or health without the service in question (this loss of health can be measured as QALYs lost without treatment, or in the absence of such data, by clinical judgment). This is relevant for identifying those worse off, thus providing guidance for the fair distribution principle. The definition of severity can be relatively straight-forward: health without treatment (Ottersen 2013). However, how this is estimated calls for normative decisions. The analyst has to decide if a lifetime perspective is to be used, which includes past health, or a prospective view, where only present and future health is considered. The operationalization of severity can involve absolute or relative measures (Stolk et al. 2004, Nord 2005, Nord 2013, Lindemark et al. 2014).

The lifetime perspective, an impartial population-level ethical perspective, implies using the health care service as part of a redistribution strategy, where the aim is that all individuals should be able to experience an equal number of healthy life years over a lifetime. In contrast, past health is not considered relevant in a prospective view. The aim is not so much redistribution, but an allocation based on present medical needs and that every patient is treated equally, irrespective of past health. This, it can be argued, is more in line with classic medical and clinical thinking. Severity estimated as future health loss translates to the clinically established expression "prognosis" without standard (current) treatment.

Other criteria are commonly seen as irrelevant (see Box 1). It is not ethically acceptable to make priorities based on gender, race, ethnicity, religion or sexual orientation. Decisions based on these criteria are unethical and often illegal. For some criteria, there is still legitimate disagreement and discussion about their relevance (for example, women have higher life expectancy than men).

Among the contested criteria, one fiercely debated criterion for priority setting is patient age. Surveys demonstrate that oncologists use patient age when deciding treatment, even if a large majority say they are against such a use (Werntoft and Edberg 2009, Department of Health 2012). Some claim that any use of age in priority setting is discriminatory and ageist (Rivlin 2000), while others argue that the use of age can be justifiable (Bognar 2008). Those with experience from clinical work know that age is often used as a proxy for other factors like risk and severity (e.g.: breast cancer screening in Norway is offered to women at a certain age; this decision was partly based on their risk of cancer). This is an indirect use of age, and can be acceptable if there is a documented correlation between age and the relevant factor (in this case: risk). Other examples of indirect use are in the allocation of organs (as a proxy for potential benefit), in treatment decisions (as proxy for physiology and pharmacokinetic changes) and estimates of survival (prediction tools like Adjuvant! Online (Adjuvant Inc 2017) and PREDICT (NHS 2017) use age as input). Overall cancer mortality is closely related to patient age.

Age can also be used as a direct factor in priority setting, having an independent impact on allocation of resources. This is not commonly accepted, nor is it used in daily clinical practice, but it may be relevant and has been suggested in some priority setting situations, like in a pandemic (Persad et al. 2009).

Other disputed criteria are personal responsibility (e.g. should smokers with smoking-related lung cancer receive less priority?), rare diseases (e.g. should we accept higher prices for so-called orphan drugs that are used to treat very rare conditions?) and innovation (e.g. should new and innovative cancer treatments be given higher priority because they can potentially lead to better treatments in the future?).

3. Recent developments in Norway

In this section, we will give a brief presentation of the tradition and development of systematic priority setting work at a national level in Norway. We will give a short historical overview, and then look closer at the process that led to a White Paper on priority setting from the Government (Ministry of Health and Care Services 2016) and to parliamentary endorsement. This will provide a base for the case of pembrolizumab discussed in the final section.

a. Priority setting history

The first Norwegian priority-setting committee, led by Professor Inge Lønning, was appointed by the Cabinet in 1985 (Official Norwegian Reports 1987). The impetus was the recognition that technological innovation called for an in-depth assessment of the relationship between medicine, ethics, and economics. In its mandate, the Committee was asked to consider five principles or dimensions: severity of disease, equal opportunities for treatment (independently of geographic, social, and age-dependent differences), waiting time, health-economic aspects, and the patient's responsibility for his or her condition. In its final report two years later, the Committee suggested that all five were important, but recommended severity of disease as the main criterion for priority setting.

In 1996, the Cabinet appointed the second official priority-setting committee, also led by Professor Lønning, to update the existing priority-setting guidelines. The underlying motivation was the ever-increasing possibilities for diagnosis and treatment, as well as an increasing number of elderly and chronically ill people. On top of this, the criteria proposed by the first committee were seen as too general and as leaving too much room for individual interpretation and judgment. In its final report the following year, the Committee proposed three criteria: severity of disease, benefit, and cost-effectiveness (Official Norwegian Reports 1997). The Committee's recommendations provided the basis for the subsequent Patients' Rights Act, priority-setting regulations, national guidelines for priority setting, and the establishment of a permanent council for priority setting in health care (Norwegian Directorate of Health 2012).

Before the general election in 2013, debates on priority setting and health policy were quite visible in the media. In particular, one case was dominant: should treatment of melanoma with the new immunotherapy drug ipilimumab be reimbursed by the state? Media coverage was intense, and in the end the Minister of Health ordered ipilimumab treatment to be part of a clinical study. The existing priority setting criteria was considered to be too unspecific, unable to provide guidance in difficult situations like the ipilimumab case (Marius Moe 2013). Therefore, in June 2013 the Cabinet appointed a third priority setting committee: the Norwegian Committee on Priority Setting in Health Care. The committee had 14 members, and was chaired by Ole Frithjof Norheim, professor of medical ethics at the University of Bergen.

The committee delivered their report 'Open and Fair - priority setting in the health service' in November 2014 (Norwegian Ministry of Health and Care Services 2014). The report attracted considerable attention and debate.

Especially controversial was the proposed method of estimating severity and the indirect effect patient age had on this criterion. Based on arguments of fairness and redistribution, the committee suggested that severity be measured as expected lifetime health loss. After a fierce debate and a public hearing, the Ministry of Health and Care Services appointed a working group that considered alternative measures of severity. Their recommendation was not to include past health, but use absolute QALY shortfall as the measure of severity (Magnussen et al. 2015). They also recommended a clearer separation between the group level and the individual, clinical level of priority setting.

Informed by the work of the committee, the working group and respondents in the hearing process, the Ministry submitted their report 'Values in patient health care' to the Parliament in June 2016 (Ministry of Health and Care Services 2016). The report was discussed during autumn 2016 and in November 2016 the Parliament endorsed the report, with comments, and with this gave their approval to assess interventions in the health care service using three criteria for priority setting: the health-benefit criterion, the resource criterion and the severity criterion. These three criteria will be considered together and applied throughout the health sector, including both at clinical and group levels. In actual decisions, the criteria can be weighed against each other, meaning if a condition is very severe or if a treatment provides a high health-benefit, greater resource use can be accepted.

b.   The chosen criteria

The health-benefit criterion – the priority of an intervention increases with the expected health benefit from the intervention. At a clinical level, the expected health-benefit from an intervention is estimated based on what evidence-based practice suggests can reduce the risk of death or disability, and improve the degree of somatic or psychiatric disability, pain, and somatic or mental discomfort. At a group level, the health-benefit criterion is primarily concerned with estimated health-benefits in terms of healthy life years. This can be measured in quality-adjusted life years (QALY).

The resource criterion – the priority of an intervention increases, the less resources it requires. At a clinical level, it is not recommended that the clinician maps and calculates all resources relevant for treating a patient. This is desirable at a group level, and all relevant resources should be included in health economic evaluations or health technology assessments (although a health systems costing perspective was recommended, not a wider societal perspective). It is recommended that resource use is compared to health benefit through cost-effectiveness analysis.

The severity criterion – the priority of an intervention increases with the increasing severity of a condition. At a clinical level, severity is estimated from the risk of death or disability, the degree of somatic or psychiatric disability, pain, and somatic or mental discomfort. Present situation, duration and loss of future health are all relevant. So is urgency: severity increases the more urgent an intervention is needed. At a group level severity is estimated through absolute shortfall – the number of healthy life years a patient group loses compared to the average loss for the population at the same age.

4. Biomarkers and priority setting

Biomarkers are considered as a pivotal and integrated part of personalized medicine. The possibility to tailor specific treatments to specific patient characteristics is attractive. This can identify patients that can expect increased benefits, reduce both side effects and unnecessary treatment, and potentially also reduce cost. However, as it is well-explained elsewhere in this book, there are also numerous challenges, including the analytic properties of biomarkers, their development, their role in economic evaluations, and their relation to issues of justice and fairness.

In this section we will put most of these issues aside, and examine the potential impact biomarkers can have on a priority setting decision. By doing this we are not claiming that other challenges are irrelevant - how we deal with and resolve these questions will in fact be crucial for a successful implementation of biomarkers into medical practice. However, to properly explore the potential impact on priority setting we will not address these challenges systematically, but we will briefly comment on some of the challenges related to the case study. The overall aim is to consider the relevance biomarkers can have for each of the priority setting criteria at a clinical and group level.

A biomarker can be defined as "a characteristic that is objectively measured and evaluated as an indicator of normal biological processes, pathogenic processes, or pharmacologic responses to a therapeutic intervention" (Colburn et al. 2001). Further, we distinguish between prognostic and predictive markers. As explained earlier in this book, we treat prognostic biomarkers as tests which inform about a patient's prognosis (such as risk of recurrence or survival), while predictive biomarkers are tests linked to therapies, predicting the response to specific therapies.

Below, we will discuss the three criteria for priority setting in Norway and demonstrate how a biomarker can influence these criteria:

a. The health-benefit criterion – the priority of an intervention increases with the expected health benefit from the intervention.

At a clinical level, predictive biomarkers can guide oncologists in selecting treatments for individual patients. By identifying those who can benefit the most, the health benefit of the treatment will increase. Patients with negative biomarker tests can also benefit, as they are spared unnecessary treatment and potential side effects that would add health loss. As the priority of an intervention increases as the expected benefit increases, a predictive biomarker can potentially increase the priority of an intervention (for individuals who have/express this marker).

Likewise, at a group level, a predictive biomarker can identify a subgroup of patients who can benefit more from a specific treatment. The treatment benefit can be quantified in quality adjusted life years, and incorporated into health technology assessments or similar decision making tools. In an unselected group of patients some may respond poorly to a specific treatment, while others respond better. For many new and expensive cancer treatments, average treatment benefits are modest. If a predictive biomarker can identify those responding better to the treatment, the treatment benefit for this subgroup will be higher. This will increase priority.

b. The resource criterion – the priority of an intervention increases the less resources it requires.

Biomarkers can be important both for directing treatment to some patients, and withholding treatment from other patients. In both scenarios, resource use will be affected. In order to guide treatment decisions in a clinical setting, patient groups must be tested for the relevant biomarker. This requires resources. In addition to the cost of the test itself, personnel, equipment and time are all scarce resources in health care.

Depending on the outcome of a biomarker test, a treatment decision is made. Often the costs of the new treatment are higher than the old, requiring more resources. But compared to treating all patients, expensive treatment may be withheld to patients with negative biomarkers and low expected benefit. This may save costs, and reduce total resource use.

At a clinical level, detailed calculation of costs and resources is not recommended. Still, physicians and others making priority decisions must take resource use into consideration. When making decisions on a group level, it is important to include all relevant resources.

c. The severity criterion – the priority of an intervention increases with the increasing severity of a condition.

A prognostic biomarker can provide relevant information for assessments of severity, both at clinical and group levels. A biomarker identifying a patient with high risk of recurrence, mortality and therefore loss of future health can increase priority through the severity criterion. Information of this type is directly relevant for the severity criterion, in which severity at a clinical level is assessed from the risk and degree of death or disability. Correspondingly, if a biomarker informs about a low risk of recurrence or mortality, this may lead to lower priority through lower severity.

At a group level a prognostic biomarker can stratify subgroups of patients with increased risk of mortality and poor prognosis. Operationalized through absolute QALY shortfall, this can be used as direct input to Health Technology Assessments and other tools for evaluating new health interventions. If a group of patients have a poorer prognosis, this gives them increased priority through the severity criterion.

5. A case study of the approval of PD-L1 inhibitors for lung cancer in Norway

a. *Background*

In September 2016, the drug pembrolizumab (Keytruda) was approved for reimbursement for treatment of PD-L1 positive non-small cell lung cancer in Norway (Norwegian Medicines Agency 2016). Investigating the premises and justifications in this approval process is useful for demonstrating both advantages and challenges in the use of biomarkers in priority setting.

For a new cancer medicine to be approved and included in the public health care system in Norway, two approvals are needed: first, the Norwegian Medicines Agency must grant the drug valid marketing authorization. This is normally done in a centralized procedure where the drug is first approved by the European Medicines Agency. Through EU and EEA-EFTA regulations, this leads to approval in Norway, usually within a few weeks. The medicine is then available for purchase in pharmacies and can legally be prescribed by physicians. This market authorization is given if the drug is proven to be safe and effective, that is to have a larger benefit than harm. No estimates of cost or other priority setting considerations are made.

The second approval is given by the National System for the Introduction of New Health Technologies within the specialist service, where it is decided if public hospitals can reimburse their costs when providing the medicine to patients. In this second process the priority criteria do play a central role and we will examine this process more closely. Information relevant for the assessment is collected and presented in a Single Technology Assessment (STA), which is prepared by the Norwegian Medicines Agency (NoMA). The final approval is made by the so-called

Decision Forum, consisting of the medical directors from the four regional health authorities and one user-representative. All STAs are published online, together with meeting protocols from the Decision Forum. However, due to confidentiality regarding pricing of medicines, information about discounted prices, and parts of the cost-effectiveness analysis and sensitivity analysis are censored.

b. The assessment

The technology assessment for pembrolizumab for second line treatment of locally advanced or metastatic PD-L1 positive non-small cell lung cancer (NSCLC) was published by the Norwegian Medicines Agency September 15 of 2016 (updated version October 10) and is available online at www.nyemetoder.no. Below, we will examine how the three criteria for priority setting are used in the STA.

As documentation for effect, the STA uses data from the KEYNOTE-010 (ClinicalTrials.gov, number NCT01905657). This study is a randomized, open-label, phase II/III study, funded by MSD, the manufacturer of pembrolizumab. Patients included had previously treated NSCLC and PD-L1 expression of >1%, and were randomized to receive pembrolizumab 2 mg/kg, pembrolizumab 10 mg/kg, or docetaxel 75 mg/m2 every 3 weeks. 1034 patients were enrolled. Primary endpoints were overall survival (OS) and progression-free survival (PFS), and treatment duration was until progression or 24 months maximum (Herbst et al. 2016).

In the analysis from NoMA, the 2mg/kg dosage of pembrolizumab was chosen. Treatment duration was set to progress of disease. Standard second line treatment for NSCLC in Norway is pemetrexed, while the comparator drug in KEYNOTE-010 was docetaxel. Despite, or rather because of, limited evidence comparing these two treatments, NoMA decided to assume equal effect of pemetrexed and docetaxel. Median follow-up time was 13.1 months; therefore survival curves were extrapolated by NoMA in order to run their models.

c. The health-benefit criterion

In the total population, median overall survival (OS) was 10.4 months in the pembrolizumab arm and 8.5 months in the docetaxel arm (hazard ratio 0.71 – all HR <1 in favour of pembrolizumab). Median progression-free survival (PFS) was 3.9 months for pembrolizumab and 4.0 months for docetaxel (hazard ratio 0.88 – not significant). In a group of patients with at least 50% of tumour cells expressing PD-L1, median OS was 14.9 months vs. 8.2 months (hazard ratio 0.54), and median PFS was 5.0 months vs. 4.1 months (hazard ratio 0.59). Health benefits from treatment and health loss due to side effects are also included in the assessment. Some assumptions have been changed by NoMA. This results in a QALY estimate of 1.28 for the pembrolizumab treatment, and 0.71 QALY for docetaxel treatment – a difference of 0.57 QALY.

In this setting, the PD-L1 test can be seen as a predictive biomarker, identifying patients that will (probably) benefit more from pebrolizumab treatment. In appendix 2 of the STA the effect of PD-L1 testing is commented. Patients with >50% of cells expressing PD-L1 had a significantly better overall survival and progression-free survival. In the 1-49% subgroup, the effect was weaker. However, NoMA decided to include all PD-L1 positive patients in their calculations, arguing that this would guarantee all patients with potential benefit the treatment (but this assumes that all PD-L1 positives are true positives, and all negatives are true negatives – the properties of the PD-L1 biomarker suggests that this is not so). This means that the PD-L1 biomarker is used to identify all patients who can potentially benefit from treatment, and not to identify those who benefit the most. Only including the >50% subgroup would increase average effect, but probably lead to treatment being withheld from some patients that could have benefited.

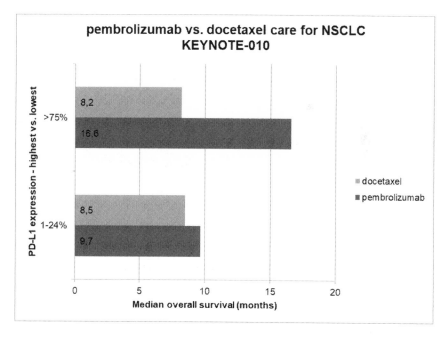

Figure 1. Median overall survival for patients with the highest (>75%) and lowest (1-24%) PD-L1 expression, treated with either pembrolizumab or docetaxel. Based on data from (Baas P. et al. 2016).

d. The resource criterion

This criterion is the most central criterion for the decision, but also the most difficult to assess. The reason is that central parts of the STA are censored due to confidential agreements between MSD and the government. The discounted price of pembrolizumab after negotiations is secret, and all calculations based on the actual discounted price are censored. Standard listing price is available, but this only reflects actual price to a certain extent. This complicates all evaluations linked to the resource criterion.

The cost-effectiveness of treating PD-L1 positive patients is 1,106,533 NOK/QALY based on standard prices of pembrolizumab. The actual ratio with the discounted price is unknown. If all NSCLC patients were treated with pembrolizumab, irrespective of PD-L1 status, NoMA estimates the cost-effectiveness to be around 1,400,000 NOK/QALY. Hence, introducing the biomarker is cost-saving for the health authorities.

There are still some very interesting assumptions and findings in the STA, relevant in a biomarker perspective. The isolated cost for PD-L1 testing is set to 144 NOK, and the cost of a biopsy to 3,030 NOK. However, these costs are too low to influence the results. So are costs related to administration of the drug, side effects, palliative care and use of other health care services related to administration of the drug. The drug price is the only input substantially influencing the final result.

However, introducing this test to thousands of patients every year requires other resources. Equipment for the immunohistochemistry test must be acquired, personnel require training, and time in the laboratory is needed. This will require that pathologists and pathology labs make priorities, maybe other priorities than they would have made without the PD-L1 testing. These indirect costs of testing are not included in the STA – something they should do to actually reflect all relevant costs.

Degree of PD-L1 expression	Effect on cost (NOK)	Effect in life years	Effect in QALYs	ICER/life year (NOK)	ICER/QALY (NOK)
>1%	626,737	0,80	0,57	783,237	1,106,533
1-49%	487,424	0,70	0,48	695,228	1,008,017
>50%	921,049	0,97	0,72	947,201	1,277,084

Table 1. Effect of PD-L1 expression on cost and health-benefit from pembrolizumab use. Adapted and translated from (Appendix 2, Table 35 in Norwegian Medicines Agency 2016). ICER is an abbreviation for Incremental cost-effectiveness ratio.

In the KEYNOTE-010 study, the effect on progression-free survival was stronger than for overall survival in patients with PD-L1 expression of >50%. This means that treatment duration is longer for that group compared to those with lower expression of PD-L1 (1-49%), which suggests that it is much more costly to treat those who have the best effect of the treatment. In terms of cost-effectiveness this means, paradoxically, that treating those who have the best effect of treatment is less cost-effective then treating patients with more modest effect (Appendix 2, Table 35 in Norwegian Medicines Agency 2016).

e. The severity criterion

In the STA estimates of severity are made based on QALY shortfall with today's standard treatment. This is in line with recommendations from the Norwegian parliament report. Absolute shortfall is estimated to 15 QALYs, without use of the PD-L1 biomarker nor any other stratification. According to the STA this is very severe compared to other patient groups. No references are given.

The potential of PD-L1 as a prognostic biomarker is uncertain. A meta-analysis by Wang et al. which reviewed 6 NSCLC studies found a significant difference in overall survival, with high levels of PD-L1 associated with increased mortality (Wang et al. 2015). However, another meta-analysis by Wu et al. showed no significant difference in overall survival (Wu et al. 2015). We submit that research into prognostic biomarkers, for the assessment of severity of disease, could provide further information for even better tailored priority setting.

6.   Conclusions

The PD-L1 biomarker influences both the health-benefit and the resource criterion, while it does not influence the severity criterion in the STA of pembrolizumab for second line treatment of NSCLC. Hence, biomarkers can influence priority setting decisions. But the question is: does it lead to better decisions?

There are still many uncertainties to the use of PD-L1. A recent comment by Vachhani and Chen highlights some (Vachhani and Chen 2016): PD-L1 expression is dynamic, and varies by time, location and previous treatment. There is no agreement on which cells to measure: immune cells, stromal cells or tumour cells – they can all express PD-L1. There is no standardized methodology for measuring PD-L1 expression, making comparisons difficult. There is considerable variability in PD-L1 antibody assays and a lack of definition of PD-L1 positivity. The REMARK guidelines (Altman, McShane et al. 2014) give recommendations for reporting biomarker studies, and the evidence used for the PD-L1 biomarker does not fulfil many of those recommendations.

In priority setting, a fair decision is a good decision. A biomarker that increases the probability of a fair decision being made is a good biomarker. At present, expression of PD-L1 is – at the policy level -- considered a good enough biomarker to be used in a priority setting decision. However, the question if the PD-L1 biomarker contributes to a fairer priority decision has yet to be answered. Perhaps it was introduced too early? The shortcomings of PD-L1 as a biomarker are many, including lack of validity. Yet, by using this test it is likely that some patients may be denied beneficial treatment, and some will be accepted for treatment without really benefiting more than with standard treatment.

It is to be hoped that both prognostic and predictive future biomarkers will have characteristics that make them better than the PD-L1 biomarker. This would benefit both patients and the priority setting process.

7. References

Adjuvant Inc. (2017). "Adjuvant! Online." from https://www.adjuvantonline.com/.

Altman, D. G., L. M. McShane, W. Sauerbrei, S. E. Taube and M. M. Cavenagh (2014). "REMARK (REporting Recommendations for Tumor MARKer Prognostic Studies)." Guidelines for Reporting Health Research: A User's Manual: 241-249.

Arneson, R. (2013). "Egalitarianism." The Stanford Encyclopedia of Philosophy (Summer 2013 Edition).

Bognar, G. (2008). Age-Weighting. Economics and Philosophy 24(2), 167-189.

Brock, D. and D. Wikler (2006). Ethical issues in resource allocation, research, and new product development. Disease control priorities in developing countries 2, 259-260.

Colburn, W., V. G. DeGruttola, D. L. DeMets, G. J. Downing, D. F. Hoth, J. A. Oates, C. C. Peck, R. T. Schooley, B. A. Spilker and J. Woodcock (2001). Biomarkers and surrogate endpoints: Preferred definitions and conceptual framework. Biomarkers Definitions Working Group. Clinical Pharmacol & Therapeutics 69, 89-95.

Daniels, N. and J. E. Sabin (2008). Setting limits fairly: learning to share resources for health, Oxford University Press.

Department of Health (2012). The impact of patient age on decision making in oncology, Department of Health.

Gold, M. R., D. Stevenson and D. G. Fryback (2002). HALYS and QALYS and DALYS, Oh My: similarities and differences in summary measures of population Health. Annual Review of Public Health 23(1), 115-134.

Herbst, R. S., P. Baas, D.-W. Kim, E. Felip, J. L. Pérez-Gracia, J.-Y. Han, J. Molina, J.-H. Kim, C. D. Arvis, M.-J. Ahn, M. Majem, M. J. Fidler, G. de Castro Jr, M. Garrido, G. M. Lubiniecki, Y. Shentu, E. Im, M. Dolled-Filhart and E. B. Garon (2016). Pembrolizumab versus docetaxel for previously treated, PD-L1-positive, advanced non-small-cell lung cancer (KEYNOTE-010): a randomised controlled trial. The Lancet 387(10027), 1540-1550.

Lindemark, F., O. F. Norheim and K. A. Johansson (2014). Making use of equity sensitive QALYs: a case study on identifying the worse off across diseases. Cost Effectiveness and Resource Allocation 12(1), 16.

Magnussen et al. (2015). På ramme alvor: alvorlighet og prioritering. Rapport fra arbeidsgruppe nedsatt av Helse- og omsorgsdepartementet [*Severity of illness and priority setting in Norway*. Report from working group appointed by the Ministry of Health and Care Services]. Ministry of Health and Care Services.

Moe, M. (2013). Kreftmedisin: nei, ja, nei, nei, ja [Cancer medicine: no, yes, no, no, yes]. *Dagens Medisin*, Editorial 21 March, 2013.

Ministry of Health and Care Services (2016). *Verdier i pasientens helsetjeneste. [Values in the patient's health care]* Report No. 34 from the Parlament. Oslo, Norway.

NHS. (2017). "Predict." from http://www.predict.nhs.uk/.

Nord, E. (2005). Concerns for the worse off: fair innings versus severity. *Social Science & Medicine 60*(2), 257-263.

Nord, E. (2013). Priority to the Worse Off. In Eyal, N. et al. (Eds), *Inequalities in Health: Concepts, Measures, and Ethics* (pp. 66-73), New York: Oxford University Press.

Norheim, O. F. (2016). Ethical priority setting for universal health coverage: challenges in deciding upon fair distribution of health services. *BMC Med 14*, 75.

Norwegian Directorate of Health (2012). *Prioriteringer i helsesektoren: verdigrunnlag, status og utfordringer [Priority setting in the health sector: value base, status, and challenges]*. Norwegian Directorate of Health. Oslo.

Norwegian Medicines Agency. (2016, 10.10.2016). *Hurtig metodevurdering: pembrolizumab (Keytruda) for lokalavansert eller metastatisk PD-L1 positiv ikke-småcellet lungekreft - andrelinjebehandling [Single Technology Assessment: pembrolizumab (Keytruda) for localy advanced or metastatic PD-L1 positive non-small cell lung cancer - second line treatment]*. from https://nyemetoder.no/Documents/Rapporter/ID2014_041_Rapport%20oppdatert.pdf.

Norwegian Ministry of Health and Care Services (2014). *Åpent og rettferdig - prioriteringer i helsetjenesten [Open and fair- priority setting in the health service]*. Norges offentlige utredninger NOU 2014:12.

Official Norwegian Reports (1987). *Retningslinjer for prioritering innen norsk helsetjeneste [Guidelines for priority setting in the Norwegian health service]*. Official Norwegian Reports. Oslo, Universitetsforlaget.

Official Norwegian Reports (1997). *Prioritering på ny: gjennomgang av retningslinjer for prioriteringer innen norsk helsetjeneste [Priority setting revisited: evaluation of guidelines for priority setting in the Norwegian health service]*. Official Norwegian Reports. Oslo, Statens forvaltningstjeneste.

Ord, T. (2012). The moral imperative towards cost-effectiveness, from https://www.givingwhatwecan.org/sites/givingwhatwecan.org/files/attachments/moral_imperative.pdf

Ottersen, T. (2013). Lifetime QALY prioritarianism in priority setting. *Journal of medical ethics 39*(3), 175-180.

Oxford Dictionary (2017). Principle [Def. 1.1], Oxford University Press.

Parfit, D. (1997). Equality and priority. *Ratio 10*(3), 202-221.

Persad, G., A. Wertheimer and E. J. Emanuel (2009). Principles for allocation of scarce medical interventions. *The Lancet 373*(9661), 423-431.

Rivlin, M. (2000). Why the fair innings argument is not persuasive. *BMC Medical Ethics 1*(1), 1.

Stolk, E. A., G. van Donselaar, W. B. Brouwer and J. J. Busschbach (2004). Reconciliation of economic concerns and health policy. *Pharmacoeconomics 22*(17), 1097-1107.

Temkin, L. S. (1993). *Inequality*, Oxford University Press.

Vachhani, P. and H. Chen (2016). Spotlight on pembrolizumab in non-small cell lung cancer: the evidence to date. *OncoTargets and Therapy 9*, 5855.

Wang, A., H. Wang, Y. Liu, M. Zhao, H. Zhang, Z. Lu, Y. Fang, X. Chen and G. Liu (2015). The prognostic value of PD-L1 expression for non-small cell lung cancer patients: a meta-analysis. *European Journal of Surgical Oncology (EJSO) 41*(4), 450-456.

Werntoft, E. and A.-K. Edberg (2009). The views of physicians and politicians concerning age-related prioritisation in healthcare. *Journal of health organization and management 23*(1), 38-52.

Williams, A. (1988). Ethics and efficiency in the provision of health care. *Royal Institute of Philosophy Lecture Series 23*, 111-126.

Williams, A. (1992). Cost-effectiveness analysis: is it ethical? *Journal of medical ethics 18*(1), 7-11.

Wu, P., D. Wu, L. Li, Y. Chai and J. Huang (2015). PD-L1 and survival in solid tumors: a meta-analysis. *PloS one 10*(6), e0131403.

5

JUST CARING: PRECISION MEDICINE, CANCER BIOMARKERS AND ETHICAL AMBIGUITY

Leonard M. Fleck

The hope of many researchers is that cancer biomarkers might prove to be especially useful for better targeting of those anti-cancer therapeutic interventions collectively referred to as "personalized" or "precision" medicine. As Janes et al. (2015) have noted, such interventions "are often marginally efficacious, toxic, and costly, so that sparing patients ineffective treatments is expected to improve outcomes and decrease medical costs." I do not doubt the worthiness of this goal. Janes et al. doubt that such a goal is realistic. For purposes of this essay I want to put aside their pessimism and assume that at least some modest degree of success is achievable. Should we see such an outcome as unequivocally ethically praiseworthy? I will argue for a negative answer to this question.

1.   Just Caring: Rationing, Ragged Edges, and Rough Justice

I will focus in particular on ethical concerns related to health care justice or fair resource allocation. In my research (Fleck, 2009) I refer to this as the "Just Caring" problem. In a sentence, what does it mean to be a "just" and "caring" society when we have only limited resources to meet virtually unlimited health care needs? The "limited resources" refers to the money

Anne Blanchard and Roger Strand (Eds.), *Cancer Biomarkers: Ethics, Economics and Society.* Bergen: Megaloceros Press, 2017. ISBN 978-82-91851-04-4 (paperback).
https://doi.org/10.24994/2018/b.biomarkers © The Authors / Megaloceros Press.

any society has available to meet health care needs. Those health care needs are "unlimited" and expanding rapidly because emerging medical technologies are what create those new needs that require moral attention. The explosion of novel cancer therapies perfectly illustrates that point. If needs exceed resources, then choices have to be made. This is the problem of health care rationing. The *cri de coeur* thereby generated by these therapies in the face of limited resources goes like this: How can a just and compassionate society not facilitate access to these therapies for patients with metastatic cancer who have no other effective alternatives? Further, these are targeted therapies that, with the help of appropriate cancer biomarkers, can destroy a cancer with laser-like precision. At least that is the implied hoped-for outcome associated with the oft-repeated mantra of precision medicine, namely, using the right drug at the right dose at the right time for the right reason. Given the extraordinary cost of these drugs and limited efficacy thus far, this mantra has the ring of a distant aspiration marred by ethically problematic realities in the present. Though these cancer biomarkers are intended to facilitate the achievement of precise therapeutic effects, the reality has been much more ethically ambiguous.

My working assumption is that one purpose for these biomarkers would be to identify metastatic cancer patients who would likely benefit from having access to one of these extraordinarily expensive cancer drugs, and distinguish those patients from others who were very unlikely to derive any benefit. A potential problem of justice exists because both sorts of patients would draw upon a social resource to pay for access to these drugs. That could be a public resource financed through taxes or a private resource, some form of private insurance. In either case social understandings or rules would have to exist to determine when someone had a just claim to use those resources that were designed to pay for needed health care. Presumably no one would demur from saying that individuals who would derive no benefit from these expensive cancer drugs, as indicated by some cancer biomarker, would have no just claims to have these drugs paid for from these social resources.[1] More problematic (from the perspective of health care justice) is a situation in which "some" chance of "some" benefit exists if a biomarker predicts the relevance of a particular cancer drug for a cancer with specific genetic features. The word "some" covers everything from a 1% chance of a very small benefit (one extra month of life) to a 95% chance of a very substantial benefit (three extra years of life). Is it the case

---

[1] One might wonder why any patient would demand some expensive drug that was very unlikely to yield any benefit. But these are metastatic cancer patients (desperate) who might have no other options and who might have read something on the web that suggested there might be an "off chance" that some drug would work for their cancer. However, I argue that such desperateness is insufficient to justify a just claim to social resources to pay for that drug.

that "any" likelihood of benefit and "any" degree of benefit suggested by a cancer biomarker is sufficient to create a just claim to access the social resources needed to pay for these cancer drugs? This is one example of what is referred to as the "ragged edge" problem, essentially the inability to draw ethically useful bright lines necessary for making fair allocation decisions (Callahan, 1990, ch. 2; Fleck, 2012; Blanchard, 2016). This will be the major question addressed in this essay.

The ethical concerns raised by our question are especially acute in the United States because we have such a fragmented system for financing access to needed health care. We have enormous injustices built into our system as it is, and these injustices will only be worsened by the successful development of cancer biomarkers for therapeutic purposes (as I shall show). Further, the individualism deeply embedded in American culture only exacerbates the ethical challenges (Callahan, 2009, ch. 6). European systems for financing access to health care are generally free of the basic injustices that are integral to American health care financing. However, European systems will still find their commitments to health care justice and solidarity severely strained by the costs associated with sharp increases in the implementation of cancer therapies precipitated by advancements in the use of cancer biomarkers. That is, Europe will be faced with many of the same health care justice challenges as the US.

2. Case Study: Imatinib (Gleevec™)

Imatinib for the treatment of Philadelphia chromosome positive chronic myelogenous leukemia (Ph+CML) has been one of the most effective anti-cancer drugs in the medical armamentarium. It is a tyrosine kinase inhibitor (TKI) that blocks the activity of an oncogene BCR-ABL responsible for a dysfunctional protein with the same name that generates CML. This drug was introduced in 2001. More than 70% of these patients can expect to achieve a normal life expectancy, though they will need to take imatinib for the duration of their lives (more than 15 years, if necessary) (Gambacorti-Passerini et al., 2011).[2] The cost of imatinib for one year in the United States was $30,000 in 2001. That price increased to $120,000 in 2016. For some patients (~30%) resistance will develop to imatinib, either primary or secondary (Shaver and Jagasia, 2014). Other TKIs are available to continue treatment, including dasatinib, nilotinib, radotinib and bosotunib (Shaver and Jagasia, 2014). But these drugs will also fail if a specific biomarker, the T315I mutation of BCR-ABL, is present. However, the drug ponatinib (Inclusig™) can effectively address this mutation ~60% of the time (Miller

---

[2] Some research is occurring to determine whether patients with a "deep response" to imatinib might be able to discontinue the drug after a few years.

et al., 2014).[3] That drug was initially priced at $120,000 for a course of treatment in 2013, but raised to $200,000 in 2016. Even in 2013, however, physicians raised strong objections to the prices of all these drugs (Experts in Chronic Myeloid Leukemia, 2013).

What would seem to be most ethically relevant so far as health care justice is concerned is that these TKIs are extraordinarily effective as cancer therapy for CML. They are not curative, which is why these drugs must be taken for the rest of one's life. In fact, many cancer researchers do not see any genuine cancer cures on the medical horizon, but would be thrilled if all the newer cancer drugs could achieve the same success as these TKIs in relation to CML. From the perspective of what a just and caring society ought to do, it would seem that the ethical imperative should be that all CML patients should have effective access to these drugs, i.e., no financial barriers. However, in the USA many financial barriers exist for many individuals.

About 60% of American workers have health insurance provided as a "benefit" by their employers. The typical cost of a good family health insurance plan in 2016 was about $18,000. Workers would often have to pay 20% of that cost. That is still a substantial cost to workers. About 25% of employers now offer much less expensive health insurance plans, often referred to as "catastrophic insurance." One defining feature of these plans is that they will typically have front-end deductibles of $5,000 for an individual and $10,000 for a family. If individuals need no health care for an entire year, these numbers have no practical meaning. That is, they cost the workers nothing. But if a worker is diagnosed with CML and is being treated with imatinib, that worker will have to pay at least $5,000 every year that he needs that drug. I say "at least" because another common feature of these plans is "tiered" formulary pricing. A generic drug might cost $20 or less for a 90-day supply. But a "top tier" specialty drug such as imatinib might require a 30% co-pay, which would be $36,000 in 2016. For a worker who earned $54,000 (the median income in the US in 2016) those costs would be impossible to pay. In other words, a worker with CML would have to settle for inferior medical treatment and only a 30% chance of 5-year survival after diagnosis. From the perspective of a moderately egalitarian conception of health care justice (Fleck, 2009; Daniels 2008) this would represent a serious injustice, given the potential unnecessary loss of extra years of life.

As noted earlier, the injustice described above would likely not occur in most of Europe. This is because most European countries do not have the highly fragmented system for financing health care that characterizes

---

[3] There are other genetic variants of T315L that will prove resistant to ponatinib (Miller et al., 2014).

financing health insurance in the United States. Here in the United States we might have a million employers offering health insurance as a "benefit." The term 'benefit' (from an ethical perspective) means that it is something "freely given" that can just as readily be "freely taken away." In addition, what various employers choose to "freely give" can vary considerably, as discussed above in relation to the consequences for CML patients. Not all CML patients with employer-based health insurance will have the same fate. Upper level managers earning $200,000 or more per year would be able to afford the high co-pays for imatinib described above. That means they would gain those extra years of life. However, another injustice should be noted here. Those upper level managers would be responsible for 30% of the cost of imatinib, which means the other 70% would be paid for from the insurance fund. All those other workers effectively denied access to imatinib for financial reasons would have contributed to that 70% of the fund, even though they would have no opportunity to benefit from their contribution. That too seems patently unfair. As the philosopher John Rawls (1971) has noted, a core aspect of "justice" is that it is about "fair terms of cooperation" and "mutual benefit." This situation hardly has the look of either fair terms of cooperation or mutual benefit. The benefit is all in one direction. This has more the appearance of exploitation. There are many more problems of health care justice in the United States related to financial fragmentation of health care financing, but I need to pass over those for now.

Oher potential problems of health care justice exist at the *social level* for imatinib-like drugs, that is, drugs that are very effective, very costly and needed for many years. I will call attention to two such problems: the justice-subversive role of "patient assistance" programs and the justice-distorting consequences of aggregated costs for large patient groups receiving costly effective treatments.

Many pharmaceutical companies have "patient assistance" programs that are designed to cover the co-payments for a drug such as imatinib. This has a very noble ring to it. It would seem to address the justice concerns of egalitarians since at least CML patients with insurance would have equal access to imatinib no matter what they earned as workers. However, this practice creates a social justice issue because this practice is intended to protect the profitability of these pharmaceutical firms. In short, even though these pharmaceutical firms sacrifice 30% of the price of these drugs, they will still collect that other 70% of that price from insurance firms that provide coverage for those patients (Ross and Kesselheim, 2013; Grande, 2012). Keep in mind that the cost of producing these drugs is typically only 10% of the posted price.

Given the effectiveness of imatinib, perhaps our knickers ought not get too twisted about the matter for ethical reasons. After all, these patients are clearly better off; they will not lose those extra years of life. However, the situation is more ethically complicated than that last sentence would suggest for two reasons. (1) Pharmaceutical companies in the United States have a free hand to raise the price of their drugs at will. Thus, for those CML patients with the T315I mutation, the only TKI likely to be effective in addressing their CML will be ponatinib. Recall that the price of that drug during 2016 was raised from $120,000 per year to $200,000. For those workers with high co-pay requirements that represents $60,000. But the price of the drug was raised by $80,000, which actually increases the profit margin for this pharmaceutical company through their (misnamed) "patient assistance" program. This is a social justice issue because it distorts resource allocation, whether in a private insurance plan or a public insurance plan, such as Medicare or Medicaid in the United States. In either case insurance rates or taxes would have to be raised to cover these additional costs. Alternatively, for a public program, such as Medicaid, a stingy state legislative body unwilling to raise taxes would force Medicaid to reduce benefits that would have consequences for patients, or else reduce the size of the poor population covered by Medicaid, again, with obvious loss of health benefits for those excluded individuals.

(2) The other social justice concern is that the vast majority of the newer anti-cancer drugs fail to even approximate the effectiveness of imatinib for patients who need these drugs. Many of these drugs will have median gains in overall survival of three months or less. I will discuss this issue in more detail below. For now, the relevant social justice point is that rational, just, cost-effective health care priorities are grossly distorted when these "patient assistance" programs encourage access to these very costly drugs that yield very marginal benefits for the large majority of patients receiving these drugs. There is equity here within a class of cancer patients, but that equity is ethically problematic from a larger social justice perspective because limited resources are being used to purchase very marginal health benefits.

Readers might wonder why in the United States Congress does not intervene to correct such misallocations of resources for justice and efficiency reasons. There are two short reasons. First, lobbyists for the pharmaceutical industry were successful in getting a law passed that forbade Medicare (the health care program for 52 million elderly) from using cost-effectiveness analyses for assessing drugs and other health care interventions proposed for Medicare coverage. If a drug, for example, is safe and effective (any degree of effectiveness), then it must be covered by Medicare. Another law also forbids Medicare from bargaining with its 52 million covered lives for discounts from the price of these hyper-expensive drugs (Fox, 2005; Tunis, 2004). Second, Congress wanted to avoid what they judged would be the harsh political consequences of making "rationing" decisions regarding health care for the elderly, which is how any limitations on accessing these anti-cancer drugs would be portrayed in orchestrated media campaigns.

Private insurance companies would also be faced with the risk of such embarrassing media campaigns if they engaged in explicit rationing of these drugs. Their solution to that problem was to encourage the very high co-pays for these specialty drugs discussed above. The basic idea was that these co-pays would motivate thoughtful (painful) conversations with physicians who would explain to patients that these drugs would likely do very little good for them, that they (the patients) should think about the financial well-being of their families and simply accept palliative care. However, the "patient assistance" programs effectively undercut the motivation for those conversations since there would be no cost to those patients. Instead, the costs would be borne by everyone else in that insurance plan, most likely in the form of higher insurance premiums the following year.

The other social justice problem I wish to address concerns the potential justice-distorting effects of aggregated costs associated with a patient population expanding as a result of ongoing successful therapy. This is the sort of situation that the health policy analyst, Aaron Wildavsky (1977), describes as "doing better and feeling worse." To illustrate, if in the United States we had the same rate of deaths from heart disease in 2015 that we had in 1985, then we would have had 1.6 million deaths instead of the actual 800,000. This is a tribute to all the medical advances that have occurred since then in managing heart disease. This is a clear example of "doing better." Having successfully prolonged those lives (at increasing substantial annual expense), those individuals as a class (and our health care financing system as a whole) can look forward to costly increasing incidences of cancers, stroke, and various types of dementia for those individuals whose lives were saved from heart disease. About that, we "feel worse."

In 2010 the number of CML patients was estimated to have been about 70,000. Because of the success of the TKIs in treating CML, it is projected that the size of that population will plateau at about 181,000 in the year 2050 (National CML Society, 2017). If all 70,000 of those patients had access to TKIs at a cost of $120,000 per year, that would represent an aggregated cost of $9 billion (out of $3.2 trillion we spent on health care in the United States in 2015 (Martin et al., 2017)). $9 billion will not tip the United States into bankruptcy. But it is estimated that there are 8,220 new CML cases each year (National Cancer Institute, 2016), so the costs for this patient cluster increase with each passing year somewhat automatically. This is not something that is intrinsically ethically problematic, given the effectiveness of these TKIs. However, as we shall see below, it does become much more ethically problematic when cancer drugs that cost more than $100,000 for a course of treatment and that yield only very marginal gains begin to "squeeze out" more cost-effective health care interventions that have less powerful advocates. If we need to control overall health care costs, and if that requires establishing health care priorities, then a just priority-setting process requires a medically, ethically, and economically rational process for accomplishing that, as opposed to permitting interest group politics and power to dictate those priorities.

3. "Precision" Medicine, Ambiguous Ethics

Though the ultimate goal of precision medicine would be to achieve imatinib-like results with all cancers, the current reality is enormously distant from that goal. Ultimately, it might not be a goal that is medically achievable. Moreover, approximating that goal might not be economically affordable or ethically defensible. If the basis for these judgments had to be summarized in a few words, it would be the "complexity" and "mutability" of metastatic cancer. Precision medicine could be more precise if metastatic cancer presented a single stable target for a particular well-designed drug. However, the biological reality is that metastatic cancer is genetically complex and that complexity evolves with progression, thereby generating multiple distinct targets and great uncertainty regarding the most appropriate therapeutic response. The phenomena to which we are referring are cancer drug resistance and genetic heterogeneity. Cancer drug resistance may result from intrinsic features of the cancer itself or its micro-environment. Alternatively, a particular drug might trigger the resistant response. Maj *et al.* (2016) write: "It turned out that some types of cancer can be intrinsically refractory to antiangiogenic therapy or during the treatment acquire resistance to anti-VEGF agents" (at 1779). As for genetic heterogeneity, it can either be within a tumor or among tumors for metastatic disease within an individual (Gerlinger et al., 2012). In either case, this makes all the more challenging determining the right biomarker that would govern the choice of the right drug.[4] How many times must *a tumor* be biopsied over what period of time in order to know that one has the most therapeutically relevant genetic biomarker? And *how many tumors* must be biopsied in order to know that one has the most therapeutically relevant biomarker? These are questions that have medical, economic, and ethical consequences, to which we now turn.

---

[4] One writer (Burke, 2016) calls attention to the exponential increase in the number of biomarkers reported in the medical literature over the past twenty years. He notes that during that period there were 768,259 papers indexed in PubMed directly related to biomarkers. Still, the disarming conclusion he draws is: "Although many of these papers claim to report clinically useful molecular biomarkers, embarrassingly few molecular biomarkers are currently in clinical use" (Burke, 2016, p. 89).

One obvious purpose for these biomarkers would be to include/exclude access to these targeted cancer therapies for patients with metastatic disease. It is ethically unproblematic if biomarkers show that particular individuals would suffer significant net harm if a particular targeted therapy were administered to them. No reasonable person would insist they had a just claim to that drug, and any physician who provided such a drug to a patient on the basis of their making an "autonomous choice" would be open to justified moral criticism.

But what sort of choices should be made (and by whom) when a biomarker such as HER2+ in relation to breast cancer is assessed? What we find in practice is that there are degrees of HER2 positivity. There are patients who are clearly HER2+ and others who are clearly not HER2+. However, this is all along a continuum, which will have a very gray area along its mid-portion with no bright line that sharply distinguishes those who are HER2+ from those who are not. Someone needs to draw that line somewhere along the large gray area of that continuum. If this were just a "lab decision" with no significant consequences for patients, then this would be ethically unproblematic. But the point of testing for HER2+ is to determine whether a patient might significantly benefit from trastuzumab. This is one aspect of what we have referred to as the "ragged edge" problem.

Another aspect of the ragged edge problem pertains to the problem of marginal and very uncertain benefits. If the bad side effects of the drug were minimal, we might be tempted to err on the side of hoping for significant benefit for the patient. But if we are talking about a course of treatment that costs $100,000 or more we would be risking very substantial limited social resources for what might largely be very marginal benefits. That suggests drawing a line at some point where we would be more confident that patients receiving the drug would benefit to a significant enough degree to justify the social expenditure. That means some patients who were marginally HER2+ would be excluded from receiving the drug because they would be on the "wrong" side of that line while others, who were just a bit on the other side of that line would be included. This is the "ragged edge" aspect of the problem of health care justice. In brief, the problem is that those excluded from the drug will complain that they have been unjustly excluded from the potential life-prolonging benefits of the drug. The likelihood of benefit and the size of the possible benefit for those patients might be small, though there "could" be some exceptions, which generates the complaint that they ought to be given a chance to benefit from the drug (as would have been the case with those just barely on the other side of the line). How should that sort of complaint be assessed from an ethical point of view? Further complicating matters is the fact that some (likely very small) number of HER2-negative breast cancer patients "might" benefit from trastuzumab (Takahashi et al., 2016). Are they treated unjustly if all in the category are denied trastuzumab? The answer to this question will be ethically complex and ambiguous, the details of which we tease out below. Before doing that, however, I will lay out a number of other varied instances of the ragged edge problem.

Much cancer research has results reported in the form of median gains in progression free survival (PFS), as opposed to overall survival (OS). I assume that what ultimately matters for metastatic cancer patients is overall survival. Obtaining timely approval for new drugs is facilitated by using PFS as a surrogate endpoint. Sometimes there will be a good correlation between PFS and OS; at other times that will not be true. Maj et al. (2016) report that with anti-angiogenic cancer treatment withdrawal of the antiangiogenic agent (due to progression) results in rapid tumor regrowth and no gain in OS. From the perspective of the just allocation of health care resources, what should be concluded? Assume, for hypothetical purposes, that this is true across the board. That would make it easy to deny future patients these drugs for this cancer because there was no net gain in life expectancy, and hence, no just claim to one of these $100,000 drugs. But what if, hypothetically, median PFS was nine months and gain in OS for 30% of the cohort was three months with zero gain in OS for the remainder? Would our sense of health care justice require that all in the cohort have access to that angiogenic inhibitor at social expense? Or would it be "not unjust" if all in that cohort were denied that drug at social expense? Or should such decisions be left to individual clinicians caring for individual patients, as opposed to having an entity such as the National Institute for Clinical Excellence in the United Kingdom (NICE) make such decisions for whole categories of patients potentially offered a particular cancer drug using as a basis for a decision medical and economic data and ethical judgment?[5]

Another provocative piece of research is provided by Salas-Vega et al. (2016). They reviewed all new cancer drugs licensed between 2003 and 2013 by the FDA in the United States or the European Medical Agency. Median overall survival gains came to 3.43 months. They note that there have been larger survival gains on the other side of that median but that these "are unevenly distributed across all newly licensed medicines, often come at the cost of safety, and may not always translate to real-world practice."[6] I would call attention, in particular, to the issue of real-world practice wherein patients with all manner of co-morbidities atop their metastatic disease

---

[5] Michiels et al. (2016) in their research note a "moderate correlation" between PFS and OS in the case of HER-2 targeted agents in HER2-positive metastatic breast cancer. This too raises the same ethical questions as above.

[6] Salas-Vega et al. (2016) also note that 30% of these new cancer drugs are also associated with no gain in OS. Their work is also corroborated by Prasad et al. (2015).

often have outcomes from these drugs that are far less positive than suggested by clinical trial results. This too is part of the challenges associated with ragged edges in clinical practice that generate comparable ragged edges for ethical judgment regarding resource allocation.

What should be the appropriate ethical response to the OS results reported above? One response might be that what is most ethically important are those patients whose OS is on the "far side" of the median. Granted that half the patients for many (not all) of these cancer drugs gained less than four months in OS, the other half gained more than that, perhaps years in a small number of cases. The claim would be that it would be unjust and uncaring to deny those patients those extra gains in survival, even if we collectively have to bear the costs of the marginal survivors. So far as health care justice is concerned, we might think of this as an egalitarian argument. That is, if anyone has justified access to some very expensive cancer drug at social expense because some biomarker predicts some degree of likely benefit, then everyone in those same clinical circumstances should have access to that drug at social expense. After all, as things are now, we have no way of knowing which individuals will be weak responders rather than stronger responders. Granted, cancer biomarkers were used to identify some subset of patients with a particular cancer who were likely to respond to some degree to one of these targeted therapies. But we have no reason to believe that successful biomarker research in the future will yield some complex set of biomarkers at the level of an individual patient that will reliably predict substantial gains in survival from this drug rather than that drug. That is a utopian mirage.

We need to grant that this egalitarian perspective has considerable ethical attractiveness. We might even think of this view as being very congruent with the European norm of solidarity. However, I want to argue that there is need for some critical ethical distance. To use a concrete example, just for illustrative purposes, consider nivolumab for non-small cell lung cancer where there is clear evidence of very high PD-1 expression (Borghaei et al., 2015; Brahmer et al., 2015; Rizvi et al., 2015;). This is predictive of a strong response both in terms of PFS and OS for at least 30% of these patients. Of course, there will be a continuum of degrees of positive response. Our critical question is this: What precisely is the scope of our egalitarian commitment? Ethically speaking (health care justice), can that commitment be limited to these patients with non-small cell lung cancer who are being treated with nivolumab? Or must our egalitarian commitments extend to non-small cell lung cancer patients treated with pembrolizumab as well, though therapeutic response might be less dramatic overall (Garon et al., 2015; Herbst et al., 2016)? And then there is atezolizumab for non-small cell lung cancer with high PD-L1 levels (Sacher and Gandhi, 2016). Drawing any of these lines would seem ethically arbitrary. All the drugs listed above are checkpoint inhibitors. So what should be the ethically appropriate response when Hirsch et al. (2016) report that "the benefit from the checkpoint inhibitor was higher in patients with PD-L1 positive tumours than in patients with PD-L1 negative tumours, although some patients with PD-L1-negative expression responded to nivolumab and atezolimumab" (at 1019). At this time, we have no way of knowing before the fact who those "some patients" will be. What then should our egalitarian ethical commitments require of us by way of response, at least with regard to the use of social resources?

Perhaps we need to include metastatic melanoma patients, and breast cancer patients, and patients with gastric cancers to satisfy our egalitarian commitments. But once we start this list there is no obvious ethical reason why we should not include patients with any form of cancer at all, as long as they are somewhat likely to achieve some degree of clinical benefit from any of these targeted cancer therapies. This, someone might argue, is what solidarity is all about. But then why should our egalitarian commitments be restricted to cancer patients, our egalitarian philosopher and pharmaceutical representative ask? Patients with heart disease or rheumatoid arthritis or non-cancerous forms of liver disease or renal disease or lung disease all deserve equal care and concern, i.e., access to expensive drugs at social expense, even if only marginal gains in health or survival are possible. This conclusion permits us to bypass the ragged edge problem and the ethical challenges associated with having to make fair rationing decisions or having to do fair priority-setting among health care needs. But this is entirely unrealistic. No society endorses this conclusion in practice.

No society can endorse allocating unlimited social resources to meeting unlimited health care needs. However, if no society can endorse such a conclusion in practice, then it is reasonable to ask where the ethical problem is. The ethical problem is that there is no public rational conversation about the problem of health care rationing as a problem of health care justice. Instead, economic and political and social forces (often using pseudo-ethical language) capture and direct social resources toward a favored health care need. In this case that favored need is cancer research and the needs of cancer patients. To be clear, the needs of cancer patients make just claims on social resources, but, I argue, not all cancer needs make *equally compelling* just claims on social resources. One would never know that was the case from the way in which discoveries regarding cancer biomarkers are presented to both the medical and non-medical public. Those biomarkers are presented as "credible evidence" to the public of "a chance to live longer"[7] for desperate patients with metastatic cancer who have no

---

[7] This phrase is actually used in television and print commercials in the United States for nivolumab (Opdivo™) for non-small cell lung cancer. Those words are portrayed in the

other options. Those biomarkers are used to identify *that drug for that cancer* "precisely." This is cutting edge medicine dedicated to saving and prolonging lives. "How," it is rhetorically asked, "could any just and caring society not provide assured access to such drugs?" However, by focusing social ethical attention on this question, attention is diverted from seeing numerous other health care needs at risk of being neglected or short-changed, especially if those individuals with those needs are socially or financially less well off. In essence, those other needs are ethically invisible. The practical implication is that rationing is thereby accomplished invisibly. Such invisible rationing efforts, I have argued elsewhere (Fleck, 2009, chs. 1, 3), are intrinsically unjust because they violate the publicity condition that is a core element of our sense of social justice.

Kern (2012) notes that less than 1% of published cancer biomarkers actually enter clinical practice. Later he writes: "Failures in marker development equate to lost resources from consuming money, calendar years, labor, talent, and credibility for the field. The volume of misleading publications raises false hopes, poses ethical dilemmas, and triggers improper policy changes and purposeless debate." I will put aside all the failures that occur in a lab, even though we should inquire whether there are more efficient, less wasteful ways of doing this research. More problematic is "successes" that are announced in prominent medical journals, along with national news coverage, that might turn out to be premature and greatly misleading. In the week Dec. 3-10 of 2016 an article was published by Eric Tran et al. (2016) in the *New England Journal of Medicine* discussing a breakthrough in targeting mutant KRAS in cancer. That article was followed by a somewhat glowing editorial by Carl June, "Drugging the Undruggable Ras---- Immunotherapy to the Rescue?" (2016) in that same issue. To quote the abstract from the original article, "We identified a polyclonal CD8+ T-cell response against mutant KRAS G12D in tumor-infiltrating lymphocytes obtained from a patient with metastatic colorectal cancer." This patient was identified as Patient 4095. In commenting on this research, June writes that "Perhaps the major challenge with this therapy is the patient- and tumor-specific nature of the T cells." (I will comment that this sentence is a major understatement of the problem.) June continues, "Although KRAS G12D mutations are common in gastrointestinal cancers,

---

form of twenty-foot high letters on the side of skyscrapers with awe-struck crowds gazing up in complete astonishment. In the print version of these ads attention is called to "patient assistance" programs that will underwrite the cost of co-pays that many insurance plans might require. A course of treatment with that drug costs about $140,000. Those programs would be better characterized as "paytient" assistance programs since their intent is only to help insured patients (as discussed above). That dulls any moral luster such programs are designed to project. See: https://www.ispot.tv/ad/AL_Z/opdivo-longer-life (Retrieved 29th of January 2017.)

the restricting allele is present in only about 10% of the population. Even so, calculations by Tran and colleagues (2016) suggest that thousands of patients per year in the United States could potentially be eligible for this therapy."

Patient 4095 is actually Celine Ryan, age 50, an engineer and database programmer. She was the focus of a *New York Times* story the same week (Dec. 8, 2016) by Denise Grady titled "1 Patient, 7 Tumors, and 100 Billion Cells Equal 1 Striking Recovery." She writes, "Her treatment was the first to successfully target a common cancer mutation that scientists have tried to attack for decades. Until now, that mutation has been bulletproof..." The question that June himself raises is whether this case is utterly unique (or nearly unique), or something that can be replicated in subsequent research for a significant number of patients. In the meantime, colorectal cancer patients with KRAS mutations will have their hopes raised and demand access to this therapy on a compassionate use basis. Is this a sufficient basis for a large and costly clinical trial? This is one place where there is the potential for a misallocation of health care resources. What if 10% of the patients in such a clinical trial achieve an outcome comparable to that of Celine Ryan, but no one knows precisely why that 10% achieved that remarkable outcome and others gained only marginal benefit? As a just and caring society are we then ethically obligated to provide this same therapy (no doubt for more than $100,000 each) to all colorectal cancer patients identified by the same biomarker, even though only 10% of them are likely to achieve substantial life-prolonging benefit? This is the egalitarian problem noted earlier.

This is the super-responder problem. There are often very small numbers of patients who are described as super-responders to various forms of precision medicine. These are patients who survive for years whereas almost everyone else in their treatment cohort has died in a matter of months to a little over a year. Celine Ryan (above) might be one of them. As things are now, researchers have no idea why these patients have had such extraordinary responses. We would have reason to wonder whether there were genetically distinctive features of their cancer that would explain that response. Research is being conducted to elicit an answer to that question. Suppose the research is successful. What then is the ethically correct response to that success? Is it that these patients alone, who, as a result of identifying certain relevant biomarkers, would have a just claim to these $100,000 cancer drugs because their care would be cost-effective? By way of contrast, if a non-small cell lung cancer patient is treated with nivolumab and gains only three months in overall survival at a cost of $140,000, then the cost-effectiveness of that drug would be $560,000 for one quality-adjusted life-year.

As things are now, we have no reliable mechanism for identifying those patients who would be marginal responders. But if future research identified other biomarkers that indicated no more than a likely marginal response (survival gain of less than three months), would that justify withholding these drugs from these patients, at least at social expense? A more concise way of asking the same question would be: Should cost-effectiveness matter when it comes to health care justice and resource allocation? This is the utilitarian challenge raised to egalitarians. It can be summarized in this way: If we have only limited resources to meet virtually unlimited health care needs, then is it not rational and reasonable and just that those resources should be used to purchase the most good health possible, i.e., additional high quality life-years? This is another example where we are faced with ethical ambiguity. Both egalitarian and utilitarian considerations appeal to us for purposes of making just resource allocations among unlimited health care needs.

Here is a slightly different example. Sparano et al. (2015) reported on a 21-gene expression assay in breast cancer. The trial included more than 10,000 women (HER2-negative, axillary node negative). The assay was used to assess likelihood of recurrence. 1626 women had scores of less than 10, which meant that they could avoid chemotherapy because they were at a very low risk. At five years 93.8% of these women had invasive disease-free survival. Overall survival was 98.0%. The justice-relevant ethics issue would be this: Could we (Medicare, Medicaid, private insurance companies) have a policy of not paying for chemotherapy for these women because risk of recurrence was so low? Or should they be offered the choice and have it paid for from social resources, no matter what they chose? Is this a situation where the ethically appropriate choice is to respect whatever choice a suitably informed patient autonomously makes in the context of the doctor-patient relationship? Going back to our earlier discussion, if we have a new biomarker that indicates this particular targeted therapy is likely to yield some level of response from this metastatic cancer, should we ignore any ethical advice from either egalitarians or utilitarians and instead advocate for respect for whatever the autonomous choice of a suitably informed patient might be, no matter what the effect with regard to the use of social resources? Eaton et al. (2016) cite Fojo et al. (2014) who note that 71 cancer drugs approved by the FDA from 2002 until 2014 yielded a median survival benefit of 2.1 months. Eaton et al. then comment "Whether the magnitude of this benefit is meaningful to patients and justifies the costs depends on individual priorities and preferences." More ethical ambiguity.

Cancer biomarkers have proven very useful in redirecting therapy with metastatic disease progression. In many respects this is a commendable outcome. But this also adds to the problems of health care justice for the health care system as a whole. We noted earlier the problems of cancer drug resistance and heterogeneity. Recognition of this problem by researchers has resulted in more complex (and still more expensive) strategies for attacking specific cancers. It can either be the case that a succession of targeted therapies is used to attack a particular metastatic cancer as resistance arises in response to each drug, or alternatively two or more drugs are used in combination in an effort to knock out several actual or potential drivers of that cancer. Again, no evidence exists that either of these strategies will result in a curative outcome. The realistic goal is to manage the disease process and postpone death for as long as possible. In other words, the goal is to achieve imatinib-like results, as discussed above. In the case of advanced melanoma, for example, clinical trials are combining nivolumab and ipilimumab compared to either of these drugs alone. Hodi et al. (2016) report two-year survival results for the combination arm of 64% compared to 54% for ipilimumab alone. But toxicities of Grade 3 or 4 were reported for 54% of patients in the combination arm compared to 20% in the single drug arm. Further, the cost of that combination therapy was close to $250,000 for one year, more than double the cost of imatinib. Further, the costs associated with those toxicities need to be accounted for as part of the price of saving those life years.

Hassel (2016) comments on the Hodi et al. (2016) research that "Reliable biomarkers are still needed to enable prediction of response, which might be used to select patients in clinical practice." That comment takes us back to the beginning of this essay and the problem of ragged edges. How much of a positive predicted response is necessary in order to justify providing these extraordinarily expensive drugs? In addition, there are the ethical and economic issues associated with the aggregation of these costs. It is one thing to provide imatinib at $120,000 per person per year to 10,000 patients. It is quite another to provide a drug like that to the 600,000 cancer patients who die of their cancer each year in the United States, or to provide a drug like that for multiple years of survival with various cancers, or to provide drug combinations at a cost of $250,000 per person per year for multiple years for a population of patients that increases from year to year as a result of survival.

A critical justice-relevant question, certainly in the United States, is whether aggressive cancer lobbyists would be successful in demanding funding for all these targeted therapies, no matter how marginal the benefits, at the expense of the just claims of other patients with other health care needs lacking comparable lobbying power. Again, as noted earlier, the highly fragmented nature of health care financing in the United States creates and maintains irresolvable problems of health care justice, and this will be especially true and painful with regard to these targeted therapies. If one can achieve age 65, which implies coverage by the Medicare program, one would likely have access to all these targeted therapies, no matter their cost, no matter how marginal the benefits. If one is employed at a place that provides health insurance as a benefit, one's access to these drugs will be at the mercy of the compassionate vagaries of health benefit managers designing or choosing the content and cost of various health insurance plans. If one is uninsured or underinsured, there will be no vagaries because there will be no access to these drugs, no matter how effective some of them might prove to be in the future.

4. Conclusion

In concluding, I will call attention to three possible options for addressing the problems of health care justice described above: a broad social process of rational democratic deliberation, a NICE-like entity as found in the United Kingdom, shifting financial risk for marginally beneficial drugs to pharmaceutical companies. I have written extensively about the potential role of rational democratic deliberation in addressing these issues (Fleck, 2009, ch. 5). In brief, if we could have a fair and very inclusive process of rational democratic deliberation regarding rationing protocols we were willing to impose upon our future collective selves with some range of serious health needs for which only very expensive marginally beneficial therapies were available, then we might have a more just and affordable health care system. In theory such political conversations are possible because the vast majority of us are behind a health care "veil of ignorance" for the vast majority of our lives. That is, we are almost completely ignorant of our own health-related vulnerabilities as well as those about whom we deeply care. However, the political climate in the United States today as well as our fragmented system for health care financing make that a utopian dream.

A NICE-like entity for making fair rationing and priority-setting choices for all would be a very good option as well for achieving a more just allocation of limited health care resources. The virtue of NICE is that it is almost entirely isolated from health care special interest lobbyists as well as being overridden by a political party in power with its own health-related ends. NICE relies upon both technical expertise, widely endorsed public values, and a degree of public engagement. For precisely these reasons, NICE would have little political support in the United States.

Finally, pharmaceutical companies spend enormous sums of money touting the clinical value and superior medical results of their drugs, which is what is supposed to justify the extraordinary prices and price increases they attach to their products. What I would propose is that their wallets should be "held to the fire" (as opposed to their feet). If their cancer drugs can yield an extra year of life of reasonable quality for metastatic cancer patients, then they ought to be paid the full $100,000 price. On the other hand, for those patients who gain no more than three extra months of life, they should be paid no more than $5,000. For six extra months of life, a payment of $25,000 might be reasonable. This sends a clear message to pharmaceutical companies that their research must yield products that consistently deliver therapeutic results that justify the prices they wish to demand from society. This has the ethically valuable result of diminishing the problems of health care justice identified in this essay. An outcome such as that would be more than marginally beneficial, ethically speaking.

5. Epilogue

I was asked by a reviewer to say a few words to my European colleagues about the possible effects of Republican legislation currently (March 23) in the US Congress to replace the Affordable Care Act (ACA), especially in relation to access to these targeted cancer therapies. Let me begin with some pure political analysis. Legislation that has a budgetary impact must be "scored" by the Congressional Budget Office (CBO). That is, the CBO must assess as carefully as possible the economic consequences for the federal government. The CBO concluded that by the year 2026 the changes proposed in the American Health Care Act (AHCA) would lower the federal deficit, relative to the ACA, by $337 billion. This is something Republicans would cheer about. However, those savings are achieved by reducing the number of Americans covered by health insurance. That number of insured Americans would be reduced by 14 million in 2018 and by 24 million by 2026. The source of those numbers would be twofold: reduced subsidies for the purchase of insurance in private markets, and reduced funding to the states for the Medicaid program.

Under the ACA individuals who purchased insurance in the private market received subsidies gradated by income up to 400% of the poverty level (which is about $24,000 for a family of four). Further, insurers could charge no more than three times the price of a base plan to older individuals who had costlier health problems. That kept the cost of insurance affordable for those individuals (age 50-64). But under the AHCA the subsidies would be graded by age and greatly reduced. An individual in their twenties would get a subsidy of $2,000 while individuals in the fifties or early sixties would get subsidies of either $3,500 or $4,000. Moreover, insurance companies would be allowed to charge five times the base price of insurance for older individuals (age 50-64). What this practically means is that these older individuals with health problems and in the lower half of our income spectrum would have insurance plans that cost $20,000 and only a $4,000 subsidy, which means they are unaffordable. Under the ACA such an individual would be responsible for no more than $2,000 in insurance cost. To my mind, this is presumptively unjust because individuals with greater health needs for which there was costly but effective interventions would be denied reliable access to those interventions. One might imagine that this would be embarrassing to Republicans. However, they are using as excusing "ethical" rhetoric that these individuals "chose freely" not to purchase that insurance. Consequently, *they alone* are responsible for any adverse health consequences they suffer as a result of their *poor irresponsible personal choices*. What also needs to be noted is that thousands of these individuals will die prematurely as a result of their not having access to needed and effective health care for what might prove to be life-threatening medical problems. However, all of their deaths will be from "natural causes," as opposed to explicit governmental rationing decisions. In other words, these deaths will be scattered across the United States and will never garner a newspaper headline. This is another instance of the "invisible rationing" I commented on in my essay and other publications (Fleck, 2009). Republicans thereby spare themselves from being held ethically responsible for any of these deaths.

The same outcome will occur with regard to our Medicaid program, which is designed to assure access to needed health care for the poor. The Medicaid program, in its current form, is a joint federal state program. The federal government will pay up to 75% of the costs of meeting the health care needs of the poor in each state. However, states are allowed to decide how poor individuals must be in order to receive Medicaid coverage. Consequently, many of our southern states cover only those at 25% of the poverty level or below. (Under the ACA 31 states increased Medicaid coverage to 138% of the poverty level.) The amount of money any state receives depends upon the health care needs of the poor in that state. It is an open-ended budget. In practice, more generous states will provide costlier cancer drugs (and other comparably expensive drugs) to those who are poor. The federal government would cover 75% of those costs. Under the Republican proposal that open-ended budget would end. Instead, states would be given a fixed sum of money from the federal government, either as a "block grant" or a "per capita grant." Over several years the actual value of that grant would decline because the dollar amount might increase by 3% while health care costs overall rose 6%. States would then have to rely upon their taxpayers to make up the difference, or else they would have to reduce the scope of covered benefits (no very expensive drugs), or they would have to exclude various poor individuals entirely from coverage (who might have an income of 70% of the poverty level or above). States could also reduce payment to physicians and hospitals caring for Medicaid patients, in effect shifting responsibility for making rationing/ cost control decisions down to less visible levels. Again, this saves the federal government money (winning praise for Congressional Republicans) but spares them from any condemnation for precipitating the premature deaths of thousands nameless, faceless, invisible individuals, all of whom would either die a natural death or suffer the unfortunate effects of some natural (non-Republican) disease process.

In brief, precision medicine and targeted therapies will be readily available to paytients (sic) who are responsible and hardworking and insured (financially visible). But the poor uninsured will be invisible, and consequently, poor targets for precision medicine.

6. References

Blanchard, A. (2016). Mapping social and ethical aspects of cancer biomarkers. *New Biotechnology, 33*, 763-72.

Borghaei, H., Paz-Ares, L., Horn, L., et al. (2015). Nivolumab versus docetaxel in nonsquamous non-small-cell lung cancer. *New England Journal of Medicine, 373*(17), 1627-39.

Brahmer, J., Reckamp, K. L., Bass, P., et al. (2015). Nivolumab versus docetaxel in advanced squamous-cell non-small-cell lung cancer. *New England Journal of Medicine, 373*(1), 123-35.

Burke, H. B. (2016). Predicting clinical outcomes using molecular biomarkers. *Biomarkers in Cancer, 8*, 89-99.

Callahan, D. (1990). *What Kind of Life: The Limits of Medical Progress*. Washington, D.C.: Georgetown University Press.

Callahan, D. (2009). *Taming the Beloved Beast: How Medical Technology Costs Are Destroying Our Health Care System*. Princeton, N.J.: Princeton University Press.

Daniels, N. (2008). *Just Health: Meeting Health Needs Fairly*. New York: Cambridge University Press.

Eaton, K. D., Jagels, B., Martins, R. G. (2016). Value-based care in lung cancer. *The Oncologist, 21*, 903-06.

Experts in Chronic Myeloid Leukemia (2013). The price of drugs for chronic myeloid leukemia (CML) is a reflection of the unsustainable prices of cancer drugs: from the perspective of a large group of CML experts. *Blood, 121*(22), 4439-42.

Fleck, L. M. (2009). *Just Caring: Rational Democratic Deliberation and Health Care Rationing*. New York: Oxford University Press.

Fleck, L. M. (2012). Pharmacogenomics and personalized medicine: wicked problems, ragged edges and ethical precipices. *New Biotechnology, 29*(6), 757-68.

Fojo, T., Mailankody, S., Lo, A. (2014). Unintended consequences of expensive cancer therapeutics----the pursuit of marginal indications and a me-too mentality that stifles innovation and creativity. The John Conley lecture. *JAMA Otolaryngology Head and Neck Surgery, 140*, 1225-36.

Fox, J. (2005). Medicare should, but cannot, consider cost: legal impediments to a sound policy. *Buffalo Law Review, 53*(2), 577-633.

Gambacorti-Passerini, C., Antolini, L., Francois-Xavier, M., et al. (2011). Multicenter independent assessment of outcomes in chronic myeloid leukemia patients treated with imatinib. *Journal of the National Cancer Institute, 103*(7), 553-61.

Garon, E. B., Rizvi, N. A., Hui, R., et al. and the Keynote-001 investigators (2015). Pembrolizumab for the treatment of non-small-cell lung cancer. *New England Journal of Medicine, 372*(21), 2018-28.

Gerlinger, M., Rowan, A. J., Horswell, S. et al. (2012). Intratumor heterogeneity and branched evolution revealed by multiregion sequencing. *New England Journal of Medicine,*

366(10), 883-92.

Grady, D. (2016). 1 patient, 7 tumors, and 100 billion cells equal 1 striking recovery. *New York Times*, Dec. 7. Retrieved 29th of January 2017, from https://www.nytimes.com/2016/12/07/health/cancer-immunotherapy.html?_r=0

Grande, D. (2012). The cost of drug coupons. *JAMA, 307*, 2375-76.

Hassel, J. C. (2016). Ipilimumab versus nivolumab in advanced melanoma. *Lancet Oncology, 17*, 1471-72.

Herbst, R. S., Baas, P., Kim, D. W. et al. (2016). Pembrolizumab versus docetaxel for previously treated, PD-L1-positive, advanced non-small-cell lung cancer (KEYNOTE-010): a randomized controlled trial. *Lancet, 387*, 1540-50.

Hirsch, F. R., Suda, K., Wiens, J., Bunn, P. A. (2016). New and emerging targeted treatments in advanced non-small-cell lung cancer. *Lancet, 388*, 1012-24.

Hodi, F. S., Chesney, J., Pavlick, A. C., et al. (2016). Combined nivolumab and ipilimumab versus implimumab alone in patients with advanced melanoma: 2-year overall survival outcomes in a multicenter, randomized, controlled phase 2 trial. *Lancet Oncology, 17*, 1558-68.

Janes, H., Pepe, M. S., McShane, L. M., et al. (2015). The fundamental difficulty with evaluating the accuracy of biomarkers guiding treatment. *Journal of the National Cancer Institute, 107*(8), djv157.

June, C. H. (2016). Drugging the undruggable Ras---immunotherapy to the rescue? *New England Journal of Medicine, 375*(23), 2286-89.

Kern, S. E. (2012). Why your new cancer biomarker may never work: recurrent patterns and remarkable diversity in biomarker failures. *Cancer Research, 72*(23), 6097-6101.

Maj, E., Papiernik, D., Wietrzyk, J. (2016). Antiangiogenic cancer treatment: the great discovery and greater complexity (review). *International Journal of Oncology, 49*, 1773-84.

Martin, A. B., Hartman, M., Washington, B., et al. (2017). National health spending: faster growth in 2015 as coverage expands and utilization increases. *Health Affairs, 36*(1), web first. Retrieved 30th of January 2017, from http://content.healthaffairs.org/content/early/2016/11/22/hlthaff.2016.1330.full.pdf+html

Michiels, S., Pugliano, L., Marguet, S., et al. (2016). Progression-free survival as surrogate end-point for overall survival in clinical trials of HER2-targeted agents in HER2-positive metastatic breast cancer. *Annals of Oncology, 27*(6), 1029-34.

Miller, G. D., Bruno, B. J., Lim, C.S. (2014). Resistant mutations in CML and Ph+ALL---role of ponatinib. *Biologics: Targets and Therapy, 8*, 243-54.

National Cancer Institute (2016). Cancer Stat Facts: Chronic Myeloid Leukemia (CML). Retrieved 20th January 2017, from https://seer.cancer.gov/statfacts/html/cmyl.html

National CML Society. General Leukemia Questions. (2017). Retrieved 25th of January 2017, from http://www.nationalcmlsociety.org/faq/general-leukemia-questions

Prasad, V., Kim, C., Burotto, M., Vandross, A. (2015). The strength of association between surrogate end points and survival in oncology: a systematic review of trial level meta-analyses. *JAMA Internal Medicine, 175*(8), 1389-98.

Rawls, J. (1971). *A Theory of Justice*. Cambridge, MA: Harvard University Press.

Rizvi, N. A., Mazieres, J., Planchard, D., et al. (2015). Activity and safety of nivolumab, an anti PD-1 immune checkpoint inhibitor, for patients with advanced refractory squamous non-small-cell lung cancer (CheckMate 063). *Lancet Oncology, 16*, 257-65.

Ross, J. S., Kesselheim, A. S. (2013). Prescription-drug coupons----no such thing as a free lunch. *New England Journal of Medicine, 369*(13), 1188-89.

Sacher, A. G., Gandhi, L. (2016). Biomarkers for the clinical use of PD-1/PD-L1 inhibitors in non-small-cell lung cancer: a review. *JAMA Oncology, 2*(9), 1217-22.

Salas-Vega, S., Iliopoulos, O., Mossialos, E. (2016). Assessment of overall survival, quality of life, and safety benefits associated with new cancer medicines. *JAMA Oncology, 3*(3), 382-390.

Shaver, A. M., Jagasia, M. (2014). BCR-ABL1 c.944C>T (T315L) mutation in chronic myeloid leukemia. *My Cancer Genome.* Retrieved 20th January 2017, from https://www.mycancergenome.org/content/disease/chronic-myeloid-leukemia/bcr-abl1/231/

Sparano, J. A., Gray, R. J., Makower, D. F., et al. (2015). Prospective validation of a 21-gene expression assay in breast cancer. *New England Journal of Medicine, 373*(21), 2005-14.

Takahashi, K., Nakagomi, H., Inoue, M. et al. (2016). *International Cancer Conference, 5*(1), 61-65.

Tran, E., Robbins, P. F., Yong-Chen, L., et al. (2016). T-cell transfer therapy targeting mutant KRAS in cancer. *New England Journal of Medicine, 375*(23), 2255-62.

Tunis, S. R. (2004). Why Medicare has not established criteria for coverage decisions. *New England Journal of Medicine, 350*(21), 2196-98.

Wildavsky, A. (1977). Doing better and feeling worse: the political pathology of health policy. In Knowles, J. H. (Ed.), *Doing Better and Feeling Worse: Health in the United States* (pp. 105-24). New York: Norton.

6

HEALTH RESEARCH MEETS BIG DATA: THE SCIENCE AND POLITICS OF PRECISION MEDICINE

Alessandro Blasimme

1. Introduction

The exponential growth of biomarker research in the last two decades has fueled the prospect of tailoring treatment to the specific physio-pathological features of the individual patient. As a consequence, personalized medicine has received increasing levels of attention. However, over the course of the years, the concept of personalized medicine has evolved and presently centers around much more than predictive therapeutic biomarkers alone. In particular, precision medicine – the latest incarnation of the aspiration to personalize treatment – currently looks at a wide variety of data, including genome sequences, high-throughput analyses of biological substrates (the so-called "–omics" data), and, interestingly, also phenotypic parameters measured through smartphones and other non-medical portable devices. The analysis and use of those data are expected to contribute a great deal to progress in oncology – the field that has witnessed the most remarkable advances in treatment personalization ever since early successes in targeting cell-surface receptors specific to certain cancer subtypes (e.g. Trastuzumab targeting HER-positive breast cancer). But the scope of precision medicine spans well beyond cancer medicine. Ultimately, many emphatically argue,

Anne Blanchard and Roger Strand (Eds.), *Cancer Biomarkers: Ethics, Economics and Society.* Bergen: Megaloceros Press, 2017. ISBN 978-82-91851-04-4 (paperback). https://doi.org/10.24994/2018/b.biomarkers © The Authors / Megaloceros Press.

the goal of precision medicine is to usher in the era of biomedical big data and big data-driven healthcare. Under the impetus of this promise of progress, towards the end of its second term, President Obama launched the Precision Medicine Initiative (Collins and Varmus, 2015).

This initiative is indeed interesting well beyond its scientific remit. As a matter of fact, together with the development of precision medicine as a scientific paradigm, the field is also showing characteristic normative connotations that are worth analyzing. To this aim we adopt a specific analytic angle drawing on consolidated scholarship in STS (Science and Technology Studies). In particular, in this chapter, we draw on the notion that technologies – far from being socially inert and neutral objects – do indeed have a political nature of their own. In 1980, STS scholar and philosopher of technology Langdon Winner famously asked whether artifacts have politics (Winner, 1980). In particular, he was interested in reconstructing the inherent politics of the technological artifacts that science brings onto the world. For Winner, intervening in the world through technical apparatuses can indeed respond to profoundly political motives. This can be understood in two ways. On the one hand, artifacts can have the purpose of realizing a specific arrangement of power and authority in a given community. On the other, technologies can demand or show strong compatibility with some specific forms of power or social orders. However, we wish to apply this concept beyond the invention, design and deployment of technological artifacts alone, and show that also scientific ways of knowing the world can be fruitfully analyzed as being inherently political. This analytical frame, we think, can be usefully applied to the study of the inherent normative drivers that sustain the deployment of novel biomedical paradigms, such as precision medicine. This theoretical angle owes in particular to the idea that knowledge and social arrangements "underwrite each other's existence," or are, in other words, co-produced (Jasanoff, 2004, p. 17). This perspective invites to look into the ways in which practices of knowledge-making underpin specific configurations of power and authority. More specifically, drawing on the legacy of Michel Foucault, scholars like Jasanoff have long been calling attention to how epistemological activities (e.g. classification, standardization, measuring, sorting) sustain practices aimed at bringing bodies, minds, behaviors and life forms under control (Jasanoff, 2004, p. 18).

In this respect, precision medicine represents a perfect example of co-production. As we aim to show, precision medicine is a lot more than a set of new methods to make treatment more efficient (by means of patient-tailored therapies). Undoubtedly, a narrative of optimization sustains the very idea of making healthcare more precise. In this respect, precision medicine mobilizes the same metaphors of efficiency, cost-effectiveness, and rational design that have been playing such a distinctive role in the history of technology (Hughes et al., 1987). However, the emergent field of precision medicine is not only constituted by scientific claims about the progress of medicine through data science. Other than that, precision medicine exhibits a rather distinctive range of normative injunctions that deserve to be carefully scrutinized. The latter amount in particular to specific imaginations of the kind of social arrangements that should co-evolve with precision medicine with the aim of making that very new paradigm possible in the first place. Such injunctions come directly from the institutions that are shaping precision medicine as a nation-wide, federally funded scientific enterprise and refer, in particular, to the way research participants are to be imagined and, so to say, socially assembled in order for precision medicine to grow. The end of such normative designs is to bring research participation into alignment with the aims of precision medicine, that is, first and foremost, to enable the accumulation of precision medicine's primary raw material: health data. Those social arrangements thus have to do with the need to create the database of precision medicine in a way that can be simultaneously efficient and socially compatible. In particular, the mobilization of such a normative framework is visible in the activities that are currently leading to the creation of a large longitudinal cohort of at least one million Americans – the so-called "All of Us" program – that will form the fundamental basis for precision medicine research. In this domain, notions of community, solidarity, civic duty, partnership, empowerment, diversity, inclusion and protection are extensively mobilized in discourses that define the way precision medicine is supposed to take shape. In this respect, precision medicine appears to be a scientific paradigm as much as a social arrangement itself. To further elaborate on Winner's categories, precision medicine is a social arrangement in the sense that its adoption "requires the creation and maintenance of a particular set of social conditions" regarding what being a research participant means and implies (Winner, 2010, p. 32).

As we will see throughout the chapter, other than promising to deliver improved healthcare, precision medicine is therefore also presented as a solution to long debated issues about the ethics of data collection and research participation in large-scale biomedical initiatives. Our analytical perspective is thus aimed at emphasizing how precision medicine entails the co-production of science and social order around novel ways of knowing human physiology and intervening in it (Jasanoff, 2004).

In this chapter, we first introduce the origin and the basic features of precision medicine. We then illustrate how precision medicine broadens the very notion of health data beyond its conventional perimeter with the aim of capturing both the molecular and the somatic signature of health and disease. Next we discuss emergent ethical issues in precision medicine along three normative axes: issues of consent, issues of inclusion, and issues of empowerment. In each domain we will attend to the way in which specific normative imaginations relate to the central theme of making data provision socially acceptable.

2. The origins of precision medicine

Doctors have long been observing individual variation in the way patients respond to treatment. However, it was not until the late 1950s, when the term "pharmacogenetics" was first introduced, that scientists started to think about such variation in genetic terms (Jones, 2013). And yet, it took another three to four decades to see this field really becoming prominent, thanks to the realization that genetic determinants of disease could not only predict drug response, but also help uncover new pharmacological targets (Meyer, 2000; Roses, 2000).

It is indeed in the context of such scientific endeavors that a language of "personalization" started to become prominent, together with the idea of delivering ever more accurate and patient-specific therapies. In this context, the first attempts were made to stratify patients based on their genotype (Gardiner and Begg, 2006). In 1998, such attempts brought a major milestone in pharmacogenetics: the commercialization of Herceptin, a drug that targets a specific subpopulation of breast cancer patients characterized by the amplification or overexpression of an epidermal growth factor (HER2).

In the early years of the new millennium, the first draft of the human genome was completed (Lander et al., 2001; Venter et al., 2001). This landmark scientific event projected pharmacogenetics into the so-called genomic era, as testified by the newly coined designation pharmacogenomics. The latter discipline finally allowed a much more fine-grained picture of the genetic and epigenetic underpinnings of individual variability, therefore further encouraging the promise of more personalized treatments (Evans and Relling, 2004).

It was in those years that the designation "personalized medicine" started to gain attention, together with the realization that its aims could be even more efficiently pursued if genomic data could be analyzed in concomitance with patient-specific behavioral and environmental data (Ginsburg and Willard, 2009). The promise attached to data-driven personalized medicine is to provide "each patient with the right drug at the right dose at the right time" (Hamburg and Collins, 2010). As those ideas gained traction both in the scientific community and in public discourse, second- (or next-) generation sequencing machines became available. As a consequence, the cost of genome sequencing started to decline remarkably, dropping from ten million dollars per genome in 2008 to only about five thousand dollars in 2013 (Hayden, 2014). This translated into an exponential growth in the number of human genomes being sequenced every day around the world. As such huge amounts of data became available, many started to consider the possibility of reading those data through a systems-based approach (Weston and Hood, 2004). More recently, the idea of using insights from systems biology to inform healthcare gave rise to the so-called "P4 medicine paradigm." The latter is aimed at leveraging the analysis of ever-increasing amounts of data on individual patients in order to improve medicine along four principal axes: prediction, prevention, personalization, and participation (Hood and Friend, 2011). The variety of data upon which P4 medicine relies ranges from genomic, epigenomic, transcriptomic and proteomic data, to high-dimensional phenotypic data (or phenome data) and to cell models of individual patients, stretching as far as to include the analysis of content posted by patients on social media (Hood and Flores, 2012). In such respect, P4 medicine, albeit remaining a research niche in its own terms, anticipates – as we will see in the next section – some of the fundamental features of precision medicine, namely its reliance on big data as the source of highly viable medical information.

Our brief background illustrates the scientific trajectory that preceded precision medicine and paved the way to its establishment. The approaches we have mentioned, however, did not emerge in any orderly or orchestrated way. Nonetheless, they contributed to the simultaneous evolution of scientific as well as discursive resources currently mobilized in precision medicine.

As personalized medicine gained increasing scientific attention in the mid-2000s, politics also started to look at it as a promising new field that deserved dedicated public investment and organizational support. In this spirit, in 2006 a "Genomics and Personalized Medicine Act" (S.3822) was introduced by former President Barack Obama who, at that time, was still a member of the U.S. Senate (Blasimme and Vayena, 2017). However, the act did not pass and three more legislative initiatives followed suite (in 2007, 2008, and 2010 respectively) trying, without success, to lend federal support to the field of personalized medicine. Interestingly, the way in which those acts designate personalized medicine over time reflects the trajectory that we have previously described. Initially, the field is described as making use of genomic and molecular data to better tailor healthcare interventions, to enable drug discovery and to reveal patients' predispositions to disease. In the 2010 act, however, the field of personalized medicine was characterized in a significantly different way. In particular, personalized medicine was presented under a much broader framing that now adds environmental factors and lifestyle to genes as crucial determinants of health and disease. This broader scope resonates – for instance – with P4 medicine that, around the same years, was starting to tap into big data and their ability to capture a wider variety of potentially relevant variables in human physiology. Around the same time, in 2011, a National Research Council report entitled "Toward Precision Medicine: Building the Knowledge Network for Biomedical Research and a New Taxonomy of Disease" also proposed that health-relevant data should now span beyond genetic and genomic data to include a host of other molecular and phenotypic measurements (National Research Council, 2011). This report, moreover, was among the first documents to use the label "precision medicine" instead of "personalized medicine."

Specific institutional needs were identified by the first three acts, including the necessity of federal leadership, the need to make discovery faster and the need to create incentives to promote data collection. In institutional terms, however, the 2010 act envisioned the creation of a national centralized sample and data repository as a precondition for personalized medicine to grow – a feature that, as we will see briefly, will constitute one of the main characteristics of precision medicine in the future. Despite its broader and more up-to-date framing, however, this fourth attempt also failed. A few years later, in 2015, the Precision Medicine Initiative took off, finally lending federal support to this field both in terms of funding and organizational resources. The framing of precision medicine consolidated the latest developments in the field defining it as "an innovative approach to disease prevention and treatment that takes into account individual differences in people's genes, environments and lifestyles" (The White House, 2015). The most prominent institutional arrangement proposed so far in the context of the Precision Medicine Initiative, is the creation of a national research cohort that has recently been given quite an evocative name: the "All of Us" program. The program aims to create a data repository from at least one million volunteers, both patients and healthy individuals, who will contribute with a wide variety of data ranging from their electronic health records to genetic and genomic data, and from phenotypic measurements obtained through smartphones and wearable devices to content posted on social media.

Thanks to the data amassed via the "All of Us" program, the Precision Medicine Initiative's near-term aim is to accelerate progress in targeted cancer therapy (Collins and Varmus, 2015). Moreover, this longitudinal cohort is expected to improve, in the long run, our understanding of disease risk and mechanisms, together with the delivery of more effective therapies (ibid.).

3. Biomedical big data and the signature of disease

We have seen so far how the transition from early pharamacogenetics to mature personalized (or precision) medicine involved considering a broader array of data types to be relevant to variability in individual response to treatment. In particular, precision medicine now relies on "biomedical big data" (Vayena and Gasser, 2016). This expression refers to "all health-relevant data that can be made interoperable and thus amenable to state-of-the-art predictive data mining for health related purposes" (Vayena and Blasimme, in preparation). Biomedical big data can be derived from multiple sources. Typically health data are generated whenever patients get in contact with medical services, but also in the course of public health activities (like health surveillance campaigns) or in the context of medical research. Those conventional sources, however, can now be enriched with environmental data revealing patients' exposure to sunlight or pollution, as well as with data about individual lifestyle, habits and behaviors collected directly by patients through mobile devices, or inferred from the analysis of unstructured data such as social medial content (Lipworth et al., 2017; WHO 2016). Multiplex (or multi-parametric) data of this sort lend themselves to new analytical methods in data science such as data mining, artificial intelligence, machine learning, and deep learning. This possibility is said to offer unprecedented opportunities for improving medical prediction and decision making (Bender, 2015).

Reliance on such multiplex data models undermines any sharp separation between data produced in clinical settings and other forms of data that do not conventionally qualify as health data. All the disparate kinds of data that can be used to describe an individual correspond to what Jain and colleagues have recently called the digital phenotype (Jain et al., 2015). This expression draws on Dawkins' notion of the extended phenotype (Dawkins, 2016) and captures the idea that the digital traces of our health and behavior "create a unified, nuanced view of human disease [and of] the experience of illness [...]: [t]hrough the lens of the digital phenotype, an individual's interaction with digital technologies affects the full spectrum of human disease from diagnosis, to treatment, to chronic disease management" (Jain et al., 2015). Such use of big data as phenotypic measurements leading to more accurate prediction of disease onset, disease progression, and treatment outcomes is at the heart of what many started to call 'deep phenotyping' (Delude, 2015), that is, "the precise and comprehensive analysis of phenotypic abnormalities in which the individual components of the phenotype are observed and described" (Robinson, 2012). In this sense, the very notion of a biomarker may also be expanding. A biomarker is defined as a "characteristic that is objectively measured and evaluated as an indicator of normal biological processes, pathogenic processes, or pharmacologic responses to a therapeutic intervention" (Biomarkers Definitions Working Group, 2001, p. 91). In recent medicine and medical research, biomarkers have proved extremely valuable for diagnosis, disease staging, as prognostic indicators and for predicting and monitoring response to treatment (ibid.). Molecular biomarkers (e.g. cell surface markers) or genetic variants and gene expression patterns provide, as it were, the 'molecular signature' of disease (Ross et al., 2000). With deep phenotyping, however, the notion of a biomarker may also start to include other parameters (both molecular and non-molecular) that may contribute to what we might call the somatic signature of disease. The latter, should the aspirations of precision medicine materialize, will eventually enable to factor environmental, exposomic, and phenotypic data into the diagnosis, treatment, and prevention of human disease.

4.   The normative threads of precision medicine

So far, we have presented precision medicine as a novel scientific paradigm. We have shown, however, that its present articulation reflects a broader epistemological trajectory, as well as a distinctive political history. Moreover, we saw that precision medicine relies on a broader understanding of what counts as health-relevant data, one that is leading this field into direct contact with other scientific domains such as big data analytics. Embracing such broader understanding of health data, however, is not a simple matter of epistemological preference. Quite to the contrary, building the database for precision medicine requires profound social adjustments that we will discuss in this section.

To begin with, precision medicine is not the first example of data-intense medical science demanding specific normative arrangements. Actually, for the last two decades, with the sustained growth of human research biobanks and genomic sequencing, the problem of making human data accessible to science has been among the major puzzles for science policy and research ethics. As those activities became prominent, conventional regulatory mechanisms started to appear obsolete. Major concerns arose with the involvement of entire communities in population genetics studies; with the difficulty in predicting data uses at the moment of collection; and, finally, with ever-increasing risks of privacy breaches and data misuse. As a consequence, the need to recalibrate informed consent procedures (Grady et al., 2015) and to restructure the governance of research initiatives in a more inclusive and participatory direction (O'Doherty et al., 2011) became the object of intense bioethical discussion. With the recently emerging trend towards using data available online for medical research purposes, those issues became even more pressing (Grady et al., 2017; Vayena et al., 2013).

When the Precision Medicine Initiative took shape, those issues were far from being settled. And yet, they could not possibly be ignored. It is thus not surprising that, looking at the documents and editorials produced in concomitance with its launch in early 2015, the Precision Medicine Initiative shows full awareness of such regulatory hurdles (Blasimme and Vayena, 2016; Blasimme and Vayena, 2017). More specifically, three themes form the thread of precision medicine's normative discourse: the role and prerogatives of research participants; the inclusiveness of the "All of Us" research cohort; and, finally, the empowerment of research participants through individually tailored health information. Let us look at each of those themes in some more detail.

a. Research partnership

As to the interpretation of the role of research participants, the Precision Medicine Initiative clearly constructs them as "active partners in clinical research" (Collins and Varmus, 2015). This notion stems from a two-decade long effort, mainly driven by patients' advocacy groups, to improve consideration for the preferences and interests of research participants (Kaye et al., 2012; Terry, 2017). The imagined route to becoming partners in precision medicine is enrollment in the "All of Us" research cohort. The latter will be populated by data freely contributed by volunteers who shall be involved in the governance and oversight of the cohort (Precision Medicine Initiative Working Group, 2015). In this way, according to the proponents of the Precision Medicine Initiative, research participants shall acquire the role of research partners. Therefore, in exchange for the authorization to collect and use extensive amounts of personal data, precision medicine offers to participants a promise of engagement. What we see at play here is a logic of reciprocity that stretches the notion of research participation beyond its conventional boundaries. Certainly, the necessity to provide research participants with more meaningful ways to express their views, preferences, and fears with respect to large-scale scientific data collections is not new. As we alluded to before, the creation of large (often national) biorepositories of human samples and data has already occasioned a reconfiguration of both the ethics and the governance of medical research. Yet, the specific ways in which the governance of the "All of Us" cohort will be organized will eventually determine if and to what extent research participants will actually be partners in this project (Blasimme and Vayena, 2016). Details regarding how this role will be implemented in practice, however, are still not available. In this respect, it has been argued that deploying this model of participated governance in practice will not be straightforward. In particular, Sankar and Parker have noted that foundational aspects of this model remain to be defined, such as defining the moral bases for asking participants to share the burden of engagement; establishing criteria for selecting who will be engaged in practice; indicating criteria for settling conflicts; and, finally, setting up the limits of engagement by determining which aspects of the cohort's governance should not be addressed through this method.

b. Inclusion and diversity

The mere size of the "All of Us" program (which aims at including at least one million Americans) called attention to another vexing issue in clinical research, that is, the biased composition of research cohorts that typically exclude women, elderly and non-white participants, thus compromising new drugs' effectiveness in those social groups (Britton et al., 1999; Murthy et al., 2004). In this respect, precision medicine is sustained by a strong inclusive narrative aimed at fostering voluntary enrollment from communities who used to be marginalized from clinical research. This call is certainly aligned with the scientific aims of the field. As we saw above, precision medicine needs to draw on multi-parametric data in order to uncover medically relevant correlations. The success of this strategy is predicated upon the diversity of the data pool that scientists will be able to analyze. Inclusivity, therefore, other than being ethically desirable, is also scientifically necessary if precision medicine has to make progress in explaining and addressing specific disease signatures and individual variability in treatment response.

The inclusive narrative of precision medicine is especially visible in the latest funding announcements for the "All of Us" program. Such announcements call for the cohort to reflect the actual diversity of the American population in terms of geography, ethnicity, age, health and socio-economic status (Sankar and Parker, 2016). This ambitious plan sets out to address a long-time limitation of clinical research – one that, if left unattended, could have a negative impact on the capacity of precision medicine to actually serve the health needs of the American population. However, this plan will have to face numerous uncertainties. As recently noted by Cohn and colleagues, no research cohort can be large enough to reflect the great variability of the American population (Cohn et al., 2017). As a consequence, decisions will have to be made as to which social group will need to be oversampled in order to ensure sufficient diversity. Unfortunately, however, there are no obvious criteria to decide which particular social groups should be prioritized, or to decide which parameters will have to be taken into account (e.g. ethnicity, age, health status etc.). Interestingly, these observations lead us to think that the diversity of the cohort – far from reflecting something like the natural diversity of the population – will rather be socially constructed starting from the priority setting criteria established by the cohort's leadership.

c. Empowerment

The third and last normative aspect of precision medicine that we would like to illustrate is its marked insistence on the idea of empowerment. According to this ideal, participants that will contribute data to the "All of Us" program will be provided with personalized medical information derived from the data they donate (Blasimme and Vayena, 2017). Thanks to such information, research participants should be able to assume direct responsibility for the preservation of their health. During the event that commemorated the first year of the Precision Medicine Initiative, then President Barack Obama offered a clear indication in this direction saying that "one of the promises of precision medicine is not just identifying or giving researchers and medical practitioners tools to help cure people; it is also *empowering individuals* [own emphasis] to monitor and take a more active role in their own health" (The White House, 2016). In this respect, the role of research participants is further re-articulated. Other than being partners in the governance of the initiative, contributors to the "All of Us" program are also imagined as end users of the data they provide. Again a logic of exchange seems to play a role in the idea that data provision could be reciprocated by the dispatch of health information to research participants.

This further normative thread of precision medicine fosters an idea of personal health responsibility that can arguably have a visible impact on the way in which, in the future, healthcare will be provided. Despite the appeal of this model, many have noticed the danger that it may lead to exacerbated health inequalities. The rationale for this type of critique is multifaceted. Firstly, people possess varying degrees of capacity to cope with health information. Whereas some may be promptly motivated by predictive information to adopt a healthier lifestyle, others may ignore risk factors and medical recommendations. Such variability may well depend on the possession of sufficient cultural capital to understand and process that information. Secondly, the unequal distribution of socio-economic resources that enable people to act upon health information in the most efficient way may also play a decisive role. In this respect, the provision of individually tailored information, per se, does not ensure that such information will be used in a way that maximizes individual health.

Thirdly, it has been noted that insistence on individual empowerment implies a transfer of responsibility from healthcare systems to individuals (Juengst et al., 2012). This may result in increasing pressure to follow medically informed conceptions of the good life that may in turn result in the stigmatization of disease. Whether or not empowerment will lead to such unintended outcomes as a result of precision medicine cannot be anticipated at the moment. Nonetheless, such risks demand special attention since this cultural shift could undermine efforts at addressing those social and economic determinants of health that form one of the major targets of present-day public health campaigns.

5. Conclusion

In the first part of the chapter, we have highlighted the distinctive features of precision medicine. In particular, we have placed precision medicine into a broader epistemological trajectory that dates back to previous efforts at tailoring treatments to the individual molecular characteristics of the patient. Moreover, we pointed out the history of earlier attempts at providing institutional support for this field. Finally, we have described the novel understanding of what counts as health data in precision medicine. Our overview has thus illustrated some of the defining epistemic, political, and material premises of precision medicine.

Against this background, in the second part of the chapter, we have looked at the normative injunctions that precision medicine is in the process of producing. More specifically, we have analyzed the construction of research participants as partners in research, and narratives of inclusion and empowerment as defining features of precision medicine. Such features, we have maintained, represent precisely the kinds of social conditions that are required for the development of the field. Moreover, they can function as socially embedded solutions to vexing issues in data-intense medical research. On the one hand, science needs those specific kinds of social arrangements in order to get access to data: in this sense, a logic of reciprocity represents the normative incentive for data to be exchanged between volunteers and researchers. On the other hand, however, also the ethical concerns that sustain those arrangements – e.g. concerns about the lack of participation, poorly representative research cohorts and disempowered patients – need the science of precision medicine in order to be addressed – namely, with direct engagement in research, with studies tackling group-specific health needs and, finally, with relevant information that patients can meaningfully use. In this respect, precision medicine represents a clear case of co-production between epistemic and normative orders.

Precision medicine, as we stated in the beginning of this chapter, is thus better understood as a complex assemblage of scientific and ethico-political scripts. Their reciprocal articulation offers novel solutions to a range of scientific and regulatory problems at the same time. Those solutions, however, also raise concerns as to the possible emergence of new challenges. In particular, we have shown, partnership-based governance models – albeit fostering reciprocity with data donors – seem bound to face serious issues of implementation, especially problems of fair representation. Inclusiveness, as well, albeit potentially addressing a long-debated matter in clinical research, will have to rely on ethically defensible criteria for prioritizing certain groups or certain health needs over others. And finally, empowerment, although it responds to patients' legitimate aspiration to be actively engaged with health decisions, might indeed represent a burden for many, especially for those who already rank poorly in terms of access to health preserving resources. These last considerations are not be taken as a critique to precision medicine as such. Rather, they invite further research into the reciprocal articulation of science and normativity that precision medicine incarnates.

Precision medicine is indeed a very promising field of contemporary biomedicine. Its successful development can lead to treatments that will benefit thousands of patients in a hopefully immediate future. In this chapter, however, rather than focusing solely on its scientific aims, we tried to tease out the multiple threads that constitute the intricate fabric of precision medicine, with the aim of showing how epistemic and social orders get reciprocally constituted in the development of this field.

6. References

Bender, E. (2015). Big Data in Biomedicine. *Nature*, *527*(7576), S1–S1. Doi:10.1038/527S1a.

Biomarkers Definitions Working Group (2001). Biomarkers and Surrogate Endpoints: Preferred Definitions and Conceptual Framework. *Clinical Pharmacology & Therapeutics*, *69*(3), 89–95. Doi:10.1067/mcp.2001.113989.

Blasimme, A. and Vayena, E. (2016). Becoming Partners, Retaining Autonomy: Ethical Considerations on the Development of Precision Medicine. *BMC Medical Ethics*, *17*: 67. Doi:10.1186/s12910-016-0149-6.

Blasimme, A. and Vayena, E. (2017). 'Tailored-to-You': Public Engagement and the Political Legitimation of Precision Medicine. *Perspectives in Biology and Medicine*, *59*(2), 172-88.

Britton, A., McKee, M., Black, N., McPherson, K., Sanderson, C. and Bain, C. (1999). Threats to Applicability of Randomised Trials: Exclusions and Selective Participation. *Journal of Health Services Research & Policy*, *4*(2), 112–21. Doi:10.1177/135581969900400210.

Cohn, E. G., Henderson, G. E., Appelbaum, P. S., for the Working Group on Representation and Inclusion in Precision Medicine Studies (2017). Distributive Justice, Diversity, and Inclusion in Precision Medicine: What Will Success Look Like? *Genetics in Medicine*, *19*(2), 157–59. Doi:10.1038/gim.2016.92.

Collins, F. S. and Varmus, H. (2015). A New Initiative on Precision Medicine. *New England Journal of Medicine*, *372*(9), 793–95. Doi:10.1056/NEJMp1500523.

Dawkins, R. (2016). *The Extended Phenotype: The Long Reach of the Gene*. Oxford: Oxford University Press.

Delude, C. M. (2015). Deep Phenotyping: The Details of Disease. *Nature*, *527*(7576), S14–15. Doi:10.1038/527S14a.

Evans, W. E., and Relling, M. V. (2004). Moving towards Individualized Medicine with Pharmacogenomics. *Nature*, *429*(6990), 464–68. Doi:10.1038/nature02626.

Gardiner, S. J. and Begg, E. J. (2006). Pharmacogenetics, Drug-Metabolizing Enzymes, and Clinical Practice. *Pharmacological Reviews*, *58*(3): 521–90. Doi:10.1124/pr.58.3.6.

Ginsburg, G. S. and Willard, H.F. 2009. "Genomic and Personalized Medicine: Foundations and Applications." *Translational Research*, Special Issue on Personalized Medicine, 154 (6): 277–87. doi:10.1016/j.trsl.2009.09.005.

Grady, C., Cummings, S. R., Rowbotham, M. C., McConnell, M. V., Ashley, E. A. and Kang, G. (2017). Informed Consent. *New England Journal of Medicine*, *376*(9), 856–67. Doi:10.1056/NEJMra1603773.

Grady, C., Eckstein, L., Berkman, B., Brock, D., Cook-Deegan, R., Fullerton, S. M. and Greely, H. et al. (2015). Broad Consent for Research With Biological Samples: Workshop

Conclusions. *The American Journal of Bioethics,* *15*(9), 34–42. Doi:10.1080/15265161.2015.1062162.

Hamburg, M. A., and Collins, F. S. (2010). The Path to Personalized Medicine. *New England Journal of Medicine, 363*(4), 301–4. Doi:10.1056/NEJMp1006304.

Hayden, E. C. (2014). Technology: The $1,000 Genome. *Nature News, 507*(7492), 294. Doi:10.1038/507294a.

Hood, L. and Flores, M.. (2012). A Personal View on Systems Medicine and the Emergence of Proactive P4 Medicine: Predictive, Preventive, Personalized and Participatory. *New Biotechnology, Molecular Diagnostics & Personalised Medicine, 29*(6), 613–24. Doi:10.1016/j.nbt.2012.03.004.

Hood, L. and Friend, S. H. (2011). Predictive, Personalized, Preventive, Participatory (P4) Cancer Medicine. *Nature Reviews Clinical Oncology, 8*(3): 184–87. Doi:10.1038/nrclinonc.2010.227.

Hughes, T. P. (1987). The Evolution of Large Technological Systems. In Bijker, W. E., Hughes, T. P. and Pinch, T. J. (Eds.), *The Social Construction of Technological Systems: New Directions in the Sociology and History of Technology* (pp. 51-82). Cambrige, MA: MIT Press.

Jain, S. H., Powers, B. W., Hawkins, J. B. and Brownstein, J. S. (2015). The Digital Phenotype. *Nature Biotechnology, 33*(5), 462–63. Doi:10.1038/nbt.3223.

Jasanoff, S. (2004). The Idiom of Co-Production. In Jasanoff, S. (ed.) *States of Knowledge: The Co-Production of Science and Social Order,* London and New York.

Jones, D. S. (2013). The Prospects of Personalized Medicine. In Krimsky, S. and Gruber J. (eds.) Genetic Explanation: Sense and Nonsense. Harvard University Press, Cambridge, MA.

Juengst, E. T., Flatt, M. A. And Settersten, R. A. (2012). Personalized Genomic Medicine and the Rhetoric of Empowerment. *Hastings Center Report, 42*(5). 34–40. Doi:10.1002/hast.65.

Kaye, J., Curren, L., Anderson, N., Edwards, K., Fullerton, S. M., Kanellopoulou, N., Lund, David, et al. (2012). From Patients to Partners: Participant-Centric Initiatives in Biomedical Research. *Nature Reviews Genetics, 13*(5) 371–76. Doi:10.1038/nrg3218.

Lander, E. S., Linton, L. M., Birren, B., Nusbaum, C., Zody, M. C., Baldwin, J., Devon, K., et al. (2001). Initial Sequencing and Analysis of the Human Genome. *Nature, 409*(6822): 860–921. Doi:10.1038/35057062.

Lipworth, W., Mason, P. H., Kerridge, I. and Ioannidis, J. P. A. (2017). Ethics and Epistemology in Big Data Research. *Journal of Bioethical Inquiry,* 1–12. Doi:10.1007/s11673-017-9771-3.

Meyer, U. A. (2000). Pharmacogenetics and Adverse Drug Reactions. *The Lancet, 356*(9242): 1667–71. Doi:10.1016/S0140-6736(00)03167-6.

Murthy, V. H., Krumholz, H. M. and Gross, C. P. (2004). Participation in Cancer Clinical Trials: Race-, Sex-, and Age-Based Disparities. *JAMA, 291*(22): 2720–26. Doi:10.1001/jama.291.22.2720.

National Research Council (US) (2011). *Toward Precision Medicine: Building a Knowledge Network for Biomedical Research and a New Taxonomy of Disease.* Washington, D.C.: National Academies Press.

O'Doherty, K. C., Burgess, M. M., Edwards, K., Gallagher, R. P., Hawkins, A. K., Kaye, J., McCaffrey, V. and Winickoff, D. E. (2011). From Consent to Institutions: Designing Adaptive Governance for Genomic Biobanks. *Social Science & Medicine, 73*(3), 367–74. Doi:10.1016/j.socscimed.2011.05.046.

Precision Medicine Initiative (PMI) Working Group (2015). *The Precision Medicine Cohort Program: Building a Research Foundation for 21st Century Medicine.* NIH. http://acd.od.nih.gov/reports/DRAFT-PMI-WG-Report-9-11-2015-508.pdf.

Robinson, P. N. (2012). Deep Phenotyping for Precision Medicine. *Human Mutation, 33*(5), 777–80. Doi:10.1002/humu.22080.

Roses, A. D. (2000). Pharmacogenetics and Future Drug Development and Delivery. *The*

Lancet, 355(9212), 1358–61. Doi:10.1016/S0140-6736(00)02126-7.

Ross, D. T., Scherf, U., Eisen, M. B., Perou, C. M., Rees, C., Spellman, P., Iyer, V., et al. (2000). Systematic Variation in Gene Expression Patterns in Human Cancer Cell Lines. *Nature Genetics, 24*(3), 227–35. Doi:10.1038/73432.

Sankar, P. L., and Parker, L. S. (2016). The Precision Medicine Initiative's All of Us Research Program: An Agenda for Research on Its Ethical, Legal, and Social Issues. *Genetics in Medicine.*. Doi:10.1038/gim.2016.183.

Terry, S. F. (2017). Turning Toward Participants in Biobanking. *Genetic Testing and Molecular Biomarkers, 21*(3), 132–33. Doi:10.1089/gtmb.2017.29029.sjt.

Vayena, E, and Blasimme, A. (2017). *Biomedical big data: new models of control over access, use and governance.* Manuscript in preparation.

Vayena, E., and Gasser, U. (2016). 'Strictly Biomedical? Sketching the Ethics of the Big Data Ecosystem in Biomedicine.' In Mittelstadt, B. D. and Floridi, L. (Eds.), *The Ethics of Biomedical Big Data* (pp. 17–39). Law, Governance and Technology Series, 29. Springer International Publishing. http://link.springer.com/chapter/10.1007/978-3-319-33525-4_2.

Vayena, E., Mastroianni, A. and Kahn, J. (2013). Caught in the Web: Informed Consent for Online Health Research. *Science Translational Medicine, 5*(173), 173fs6–173fs6. Doi:10.1126/scitranslmed.3004798.

Venter, J. C., Adams, M. D., Myers, E. W., Li, P. W., Mural, R. J., Sutton, G. G., Smith, H. O., Yandell, M., Evans, C. A. and Holt, R. A. (2001). The Sequence of the Human Genome. *Science, 291*(5507), 1304–51.

Weston, A. D., and Hood, L. (2004). Systems Biology, Proteomics, and the Future of Health Care: Toward Predictive, Preventative, and Personalized Medicine. *Journal of Proteome Research, 3*(2), 179–96. Doi:10.1021/pr0499693.

"WHO | The Health Data Ecosystem and Big Data." 2017. *WHO.* http://www.who.int/ehealth/resources/ecosystem/en/. Retrieved March 8, 2017.

Winner, L. (1980). Do Artifacts Have Politics? *Daedalus, 109*(1), 121–36.

Winner, L. (2010). *The Whale and the Reactor: A Search for Limits in an Age of High Technology.* Chicago, IL: University of Chicago Press.

The White House (2015). Fact Sheet: President Obama's Precision Medicine Initiative. https://www.whitehouse.gov/the-press-office/2015/01/30/fact-sheet-president-obama-s-precision-medicine-initiative Retrieved March 8, 2017.

The White House (2016). Remarks by the President in Precision Medicine Panel Discussion. https://www.whitehouse.gov/the-press-office/2016/02/25/remarks-president-precision-medicine-panel-discussion Retrieved March 8, 2017.

7

PERSONALISED MEDICINE AND THE EVOLUTION OF NEW CONCEPTS OF HEALTH

Caroline Engen

1. Future imaginaries fuelled by the progressive precision within the field of medicine

Gradually and with subtlety, increased precision is introduced to oncological practice, one new diagnostic test, novel biomarker, or innovative therapeutic compound at a time. This progress represents significant promise for improvements for cancer patient outcome, and for the management of the oncological healthcare services as a whole. The development is however also characterised by the emergence of new challenges, as highlighted by the various authors of this book. The arguments brought forward throughout the various chapters stretch across a broad field of social domains and involve a multitude of societal actors. The range and diversity of questions raised reminds us about the vast surface of convergence between the science of cancer biomarkers and society at large. As novel biomarkers and technology are ever more swiftly translated and implemented into clinical practice, the accumulation of minor advancements cause greater drifts between interfacing sectors, generating anticipation and visions of where this development as a general trend will carry us, and what possibilities it might offer us.

Imagine a world where biomarkers are not only applied as targeted tools

Anne Blanchard and Roger Strand (Eds.), *Cancer Biomarkers: Ethics, Economics and Society.* Bergen: Megaloceros Press, 2017. ISBN 978-82-91851-04-4 (paperback). https://doi.org/10.24994/2018/b.biomarkers © The Authors / Megaloceros Press.

to assess certain specific questions, but are employed as a systematic approach, delineating an innovative way of life. This is in part the promise and prospect of "personalised medicine", one of the most prominent visions, built on the current ravishing advances of biomarker science and biotechnology. 4P medicine, maybe the most elaborate vision of personalised medicine, was put forward by Leroy Hood, the President and Co-founder of the Institute for Systems Biology, already in 2004 (Weston and Hood, 2004). In this vision the healthcare sector of the future is grounded in active user Participation, and sharing of "big data", enabling personalised Prediction, personalised Prevention, and Personalised therapeutic strategies. Composite biomarkers, derived from encompassing "omic" systems approaches, supplemented by pervasively collected digital data points describing our environment and interactions, will map our genotype and will continually assess fluctuations in our dynamic and interchanging phenotype, providing us with insight about our presence and our possible futures. This approach is by many believed to enable timely and precise preventive and therapeutic measures. The leading hypothesis is that this novel strategy will support and empower us to live healthier, better, and longer lives.

Compared to the medical services provided to most populations today, this shift not only represents a natural progress of how we think about medical interventions, but also denotes a change in our medical paradigm. Unquestionably such a commotion will cause widespread waves of effects that will far transcend the field of medicine itself, and it is far from self-evident that it will provide merely the promised advantages envisioned. There may be collateral effects, providing both unforeseen benefits and harms, which are both substantial and relevant (Hunter, 2016; Jameson and Longo, 2015; Mirnezami et al., 2012). The multitude and magnitude of contact points between medicine and society far exceed the reach of our conventional measuring stick. The gravity and extent of such unanticipated transformations therefore remain rather obscure. Our vision is additionally clouded by the fact that we are currently located somewhere in the midst of the process, leading up to such a change. We are living, researching, and practicing medicine, in an era characterised by vast and speedily techno-scientific development that has already gained a pervasive grip on most arenas of human life. Medical research and medical practice is hence increasingly supported and dependent on digital technology, computational algorithms, automation and connectivity (Elenko et al., 2015). The movement towards a new medical paradigm is enabled and encouraged by exactly this gradual absorption and adaptation of these medical strategies. As the complexity of the services provided is continuously increasing, science and technology cooperatively mould our sociocultural context. Together they gradually reshape how we think about health and healthcare, as the boundaries and limits of what is conceivable and even thought desirable are continuously expanding.

Based on my dual role as a physician and a cancer researcher I find myself profoundly vested in the concept of health professionally. Simultaneously I share the destiny of all mortals, a destiny characterised by an inevitable vulnerability to health impairment, suffering and death. Expectantly with most of my life still ahead of me I am therefore deeply curious about the impact of the shifts in our understanding of health. It seems clear to me that this process will influence and alter both various professional spaces and private arenas in numerous ways. Although vague and ambiguous, the influence and impact of these movements should consequently not be swept away as miniscule or irrelevant. The field of medicine is located in close proximity to the centre of core human values and goals, like health, well-being and human flourishing (Constitution of the World Health Organization, 1946). It is our self-perspective and our identity that is at stake: both how we perceive ourselves as individuals and as a species. In this following chapter, mindful that the shift has already been initiated, some of the possible ramifications of a change in our medical paradigm will be attempted to be explored, focusing on how the concept of health might gradually evolve. Ultimately the hypothesis of personalised medicine facilitating healthier, better, and longer lives will be deliberated, questioning the validity of this hypothesis, and reflecting on the risks we are facing, facilitating such a change in medical practice based on an as of yet invalidated hypothesis.

2. Cancer biomarkers, precision oncology and personalised medicine

To frame the discussion of how cancer biomarkers, precision oncology and personalised medicine relate to each other and to the world we live in, we turn briefly to the narrative of the cancer biomarker field, focusing on how it serves as a prominent strategy in the so-called "war on cancer", and how it may substantiate the ideas and visions of personalised medicine.

Appreciating the events and the societal currents setting the stage for the cancer biomarker field requires us to throw a brief glance backwards in history. The 20th century was marked by remarkable advancements within the fields of public health and medicine. Not unexpectedly however, as the boundaries for human life gradually have moved into old age, new societal and medical challenges have materialised. New health "threats" have emerged and spread fear and anguish. Never before has such a large part of the global population been elderly, and never before have so many humans suffered death related to age-associated conditions like cardiovascular events, the end-stages of chronic degenerative diseases or cancer (Roser,

2016). Especially the latter, cancer, has emerged as a gloomy opponent, initially offering little hope of recovery if you were diagnosed, associated with aggressive and devastating treatments like mutilating surgery and chemotherapy, and often coupled with great physical suffering in its final stages. The terror it represents is attenuated by the fact that it was, and still is, an increasing health problem globally, initially most pronounced in high income countries, but as more and more countries have emerged from poverty, also in the developing world (Stewart and Wild, 2014).

As a response to the emerging threat of cancer, 'The National Cancer Act of 1971' was launched by the US Congress and signed into law by President Nixon on December 23 1971. The commitment to "conquering this dread disease" as Nixon put it, marked a pivotal historical shift in priority, firstly politically and consequently within the fields of medical research and medical practice, and the act is often referred to as the initiation of the 'war on cancer'. Although initially a political incentive, the 'cancer war' gradually came to influence most sectors and layers of Western societies. Through shifts in priorities, reallocation of financial and human resources, alterations and expansion of infrastructure and technological boundaries, and ultimately through communication in media and popular culture, the 'cancer war' has progressively become virtually a part of western collective identity (Patterson, 1988).

The various contestants in the 'cancer war' play different roles on the battlefield, and contribute with their resources and competence in numerous ways. While healthcare providers fight cancer directly in close collaboration with the patients, the actual strategies of combat are historically refined and executed at large by the medical research community. One of the most fundamental steps confronting the threat of cancer has been through thorough portrayal of the enemy, deciphering the secrets of cancer. Identification and characterization of biological markers specific to cancer biology has been one of our leading approaches, denoting the birth of the cancer biomarker field. During the last 45 years the field has developed vastly, and its joint efforts have resulted in remarkable progress in our biological understanding of cancer: including the underlying aetiology of carcinogenesis, intrinsic and extrinsic risk factors for cancer development, and the common "hallmarks" of malignant cells (Hanahan and Weinberg, 2000). The field has gradually progressed further and discovered how we can exploit the knowledge of cancer biomarkers, not only in the preparation for war, but also at the forefront, where we fight cancer face on, predicting, preventing and treating the disease (Collins et al., 2017). The overall goal of cancer biomarker research today is therefore guided by objectives that far exceed the utility of cancer biomarkers in enforcing our biological understanding of the disease, and it has consequently developed from a biomedical field of research to a translational and clinical science (Wagner and Srivastava, 2012).

One of the significant lessons learned early on was that all tumours are unique entities, which differ substantially from patient to patient. Biomarkers can serve as clinical tools assessing this diversity throughout the various stages of the disease. Some biomarkers can accurately predict the risk for cancer development, enabling initiation of appropriate preventive measures. Clinical application of cancer biomarkers can also facilitate early diagnosis, by reviling either a premalignant or a subclinical process, allowing prompt clinical intervention, increasing the possibility for a favourable outcome. Use of cancer biomarkers also refine our ability to classify cancers through stratification and prognostication, guiding and improving clinical management. Based on individual baseline variability and disease specific features, cancer biomarkers can also facilitate therapy guidance, by aiding choice of therapeutic strategy, optimization of treatment intensity, therapy surveillance, and screening for minimal residual disease or disease recurrence (Chatterjee and Zetter, 2005).

The understanding of the inter-individual heterogeneity and the clinical adaptation of this diversity through a systematic use of cancer biomarkers as determinants for clinical decisions form the foundation of precision oncology, a therapeutic strategy created to encompass our deepened comprehension of cancer biology. The rationale is based on reducing therapeutic algorithms from a heterogeneous group of individuals to a distinct disease management, recognising that every cancer patient is unique and requires individual assessment. The concept of precision oncology is further supported by the recognition of specific molecular aberrancies that appear to be the principal and necessary drivers of certain malignant processes. Intensive focus has been devoted to the objective of identifying cancer specific aberrancies that discriminates well towards healthy cells. The development of therapeutic compounds specifically aiming at such targets, often designated targeted therapies, is one of the main contributions of the cancer biomarker field (Weinstein, 2002). This strategy has demonstrated very successful in definite cancers, exemplified by tyrosine kinase inhibitor treatment in BCR-ABL positive chronic myeloid leukaemia (Druker et al., 2001), all-trans-retinoic-acid in PML-RARA positive acute promyelocytic leukaemia (Mandelli et al., 1997) and treatment with trastuzumab in HER2 positive breast cancer patients (Slamon et al., 2001).

Although precision oncology and targeted therapy denotes revolutionising advances within these definite cancers, 15 years after the approval of the first generation tyrosine kinase inhibitors in chronic myeloid leukaemia we have few other comparable success stories to show for. The preliminary results are on the contrary rather sobering. We are currently more or less unable to provide enduring disease free responses and much less curative treatment regimens, and our combat against the vast majority of human malignancies in advanced stages remains unsettled (Prasad et al., 2016).

The lack of realization of precision oncology's postulated potential has obliged us to seek explanations for the obvious failure. Accelerated by the massive progress within the field of tumour genetics we have just lately commenced to comprehend the vast extent of intra-individual diversity of tumour cells, as well as their temporal plasticity (McGranahan and Swanton, 2017). Further multiplicity is increasingly recognised by the intricate interplay between cancer cells and their microenvironment. Through mechanisms of tissue disruption, manipulation and reprogramming cancer cells are capable of recruiting surrounding cellular elements, like various types of immune cells and cellular components of the vascular bed and the connective tissue, to join forces in their malice (Hanahan and Weinberg, 2011). This recollection poses a serious challenge to the rather simple and linear battle plan of precision oncology and targeted therapy, and explains partially some of the strategies' failures. We have slowly come to realise that cancer is a more resilient opponent than initially envisioned. Depicted by adaptive and evasive potential it is increasingly difficult to imagine that a single novel therapeutic strategy, still undiscovered, will efficiently turn the conflict of war in our favour (Tannock and Hickman, 2016).

This realisation has however, seemingly as of yet, not robbed us of hope. Conversely, we contest with ever more endeavour, resources and determination as new strategies combating cancer are advancing (Hanahan, 2014; Collins et al., 2017). From the ashes of the burning dream of precision oncology rises the idea of personalised medicine. While precision oncology tackles cancer face on, the basic strategy of personalised or precision medicine is to retract from the front lines and apply a more general preventive tactic, contrasting the reaction based approach characterising conventional medicine today. This strategy foresees vast and encompassing benefits, by not only addressing cancer but also most other health threats, long before they even appear. Born a dream, serving a solution to the failures of precision oncology, personalised medicine has quickly developed into a strong and appealing hypothesis, which currently resonates loudly and with substantial strength both in the public, and among political institutions and funding bodies, as illustrated by massive investments in European (Marx, 2015), North American (Collins and Varmus, 2015), and Asian 'precision medicine programs' (Cyranoski, 2016), in addition to the establishment of international projects like 'The Global Alliance for Genomics and Health' (Global Alliance for Genomics and Health, 2016).

3. Is it plausible that increased resolution unintentionally promotes reduced dimensionality, medicalisation and confusion?

The narrative of cancer biomarkers, precision oncology and personalised medicine demonstrates that as concepts and ideas the three of them are tightly interconnected both in history and politics. They are all built on a gradual increase in biological understanding of cancer, and they all represent an attempt to apply this knowledge in a solution-based manner as applied medicine. While neither of them as of yet have provided a solution to the 'war on cancer' the mobilisation of vast resources, of both economical and intellectual character, has resulted in huge breakthroughs in our conceptual understanding of not only carcinogenesis but also everything living. How cancer biomarkers and personalised medicine relate to health and cancer related health impairment therefore reaches far beyond the delineation of cancer as strictly pathological processes. The field of cancer biomarkers ultimately contributes in shaping not only oncological practices, but also values, prioritisations and politics.

The study of cancer biomarkers descends from the tradition of biomedicine, where non-disease and disease are understood and studied as endpoints of a bipolar one-dimensional structure. Demarcation of disease and non-disease is defined in a rigorous molecular-biological appreciation, marking disease as strict somatic pathological entities. Through methodological reductionism this approach has aided the comprehension of the natural history of human malignancies by identification of initial and characterising signs of carcinogenesis. This has increased the feasibility of early detection of pathological processes and the precision in outlining non-cancerous versus cancerous tissue. As our body of knowledge about cancer biology has gained weight, our understanding of cancer as a pathological process has become ever clearer and well defined. The methodology and the technology developed to assess cancer have simultaneously greatly benefitted and improved the sensitivity and specificity of determining and defining non-malignant pathological processes, contributing substantially to the vast development and success of modern medicine.

As the biomarker field has progressed towards becoming a translational and clinical discipline however, it has brought with it its intrinsic set of approaches and methodologies, gradually diffusing some of its values to clinical practice. One of the challenges with this transition is that non-disease and disease are not true dichotomies, but rather dynamic processes moving on a continuing spectrum. As our measuring stick becomes ever more precise and the units we consider relevant ever smaller, the stringent understanding of what is habitual and what is deviating from this baseline tends to promote an inclination for moving the cut-off of what we consider pathological, continuously narrowing down the spectrum of what is normal and healthy (Welch and Black, 2010). Health is however traditionally not defined by the absence of disease alone (Constitution of the World Health Organization, 1946) and the impact of cancer as a health threat far exceeds the boundaries of the physical tumour and spans into both psychological and social arenas. The health impairment caused by cancer consequently includes not only elements of physical suffering but also emotional and social torment (Breitbart and Alici, 2009).

The dangers of biomedical reductionism are particularly present in situations where pathology is not coupled with a subjective experience of illness, as is the situation when attempting to predict the onset of disease or to identify asymptomatic pathological processes. Both cancer biomarkers and precision oncology are deeply vested in this field, hypothesising that early detection will prove beneficial to cancer patient outcome. Prediction and early detection of cancer through extensive use of biomarkers might ultimately result in reduced tumour volume, reduced incidence of clinically mutilating disease and reduced cancer-related mortality. It is however also possible that we occasionally overestimate the benefits of prediction and early detection (Gøtzsche and Jorgensen, 2013; Ilic et al., 2013). We might also misjudge the potential and implementation capacity of customised behavioural recommendations (Meader et al., 2017). Correspondingly curing cancer, defined by eradication of all cancerous cells, might not always provide the benefit it intuitively promises. A cure does not at all guarantee a full recovery, characterised by reestablishment of health and functioning. A resection of a confined tumour might therefore cure cancer, but it potentially leaves the body mutilated and reduced by biomedical definition. The lack of recovery might even serve greater harm than the disease itself, if the condition initially was indolent and manageable (Brodersen et al., 2014). Managing cancer in a clinical setting is not only about obtaining a cure but also about providing care, enabling the restoration of function, self-worth, confidence, and motivation. In the light of novel technological possibilities it is imperative that we do not become oblivious to the increased emotional and social stress a pronounced articulated risk of cancer or a cancer diagnosis means to individuals, and the consequent health impairment it might cause. The net effect might eventually be that we unintentionally increase the health impairment caused by cancer rather than decreasing it.

The promises of personalised medicine dismantles the coupling of disease and illness even further, founded on the belief that all deviation from "wellbeing" could potentially be quantified by biomedical methods. The visionaries of personalised medicine promote strong statements on how the implementation of this medical paradigm will change our healthcare sector from a reactive institution focusing on damage control, to a more holistic way of health promotion and disease prevention in healthy individuals. The hypothesis is that focusing on prevention and early detection will ultimately reduce the need for reactive measures. Although the advocates of personalised medicine often present the approach as a backlash pointed directly at reductionism (Institute for Systems Biology, 2017), the idea might not truly retract towards a more holistic view in a traditional sense. It might rather advance by bringing reductionism and bio-medicalisation one step further, promoting a ubiquitous "medicalisation of life itself", where the reductionist approach of medicine becomes an encompassing way of life rather than a tool supporting medical decision making (Vogt et al., 2016). The hazard is that such a strategy will produce new experiences of illness and sickness that have important and harmful implications both on a subjective and a societal level, contributing to increased and harmful bio-medicalisation, and a shift in focus on cancer or other pathological processes as health hazards to threats of normal tissue homeostasis.

Together cancer biomarkers, precision oncology and personalised medicine represent a powerful and intangible force, continuously shaping the terrain they run through, imposing a pronounced impact on the field of oncology and medicine, opening up new spaces of possibilities and moving boundaries. The relationship between the field of cancer biomarkers and society is however not a unilateral one, and what society does to the field of cancer biomarkers and why, are equally, if not even more interesting questions. To assess the factual impact and possible harm of reductionism and bio-medicalisation we must turn to the various stakeholders enhancing their force, and the world in which these concepts and visions are ultimately implemented.

The vast progress we have witnessed within the fields of medicine is largely thanks to the coproduction of development through an interlaced techno-scientific collaboration where the life sciences and the life science related industry have cooperatively generated a vast amount of physiological and medical knowledge and technology that we all can potentially benefit from. The various troops constituting the composite anti-cancer force is therefore not limited to cancer researchers, healthcare providers and healthcare delivery systems, but includes also the life-science industry, policymakers and national and international regulators. The general public are also important contributors, as most individuals are affected by the destructions of cancer in one way or another, either as patients themselves, or as next of kin. Ultimately it is the collective effort of all of these stakeholders that power the force and direction of warfare.

Steadily as time has progressed, the depth of investment of these various participants has augmented. Millions of dollars have been devoted to the cause, entire fields of research have been established, thousands of careers and professional identities have been built, and new cultures have evolved. Novel relationships of collaboration and dependency have been founded, and comparable to the field of biology, these interactions are often sophisticated in character, recognised by reciprocal regulations patterns, including both negative and positive feedback loops.

As the intricacy of relations expand, our understanding and control of the underlying mechanisms decline. The current associations and interactions between life science scholars, academic institutions, clinical practitioners, healthcare delivery systems, the biomedical and biotechnological industry, political systems and regulatory bodies are ambiguous, and the power and impact of each stakeholder's objective is hard to quantify. Confronted with this complexity of interests it might be plausible that the motives and objectives represented do not always align with an overall aim of promoting "the highest attainable standard of health", the united international goal of healthcare services and healthcare research (Constitution of the World Health Organization, 1946).

One of the principal premises for the improvements achieved across the cancer field is financial investment supporting not only academic research and healthcare delivery systems, but also the private sector, enabling product development of both technical and pharmaceutical character. Commercial interests occasionally align with human aspiration for health and happiness, but poorly regulated market powers do not truly take human values into consideration. Ultimately, the only truth the market knows is profit, generated through increased consumption and establishment of new markets. Capitalism does not care if the focus in medicine is shifted from prevention to early detection, from cure to disease stabilization, or from disease stabilization to palliative care. Capitalistic powers do however recognize the unexploited potential of commercialising life and death, and the probable revenues associated with encompassing and recourse demanding strategies like precision oncology and personalised medicine. The commitment to these strategies is enhanced by the strength of professionalism, status and expertise built up by healthcare professionals and researchers deeply invested in these strategies. A general tendency of techno-scientific and innovative optimism further shades the biomedical research establishments and their communication channels, possibly creating a culture of systematic knowledge bias. Among the public, the biomedical model has also steadily gained sound footing and support, as the investments in the 'war on cancer' produces high expectations for returns in the form of better care. Promoted by a language of consumerism directed at the general public, there is a general tendency towards a conviction that the quantity of healthcare services is a good measure of the quality, where the healthcare service delivered entails an intrinsic benefit, almost completely detached of the health advantage provided. Competing interests do not always constitute a constructive force, and economic interest, vested recourses, uncritical optimism towards techno-scientific innovation and inaccurate knowledge transmission are all among recognised drivers of poor medical care, often associated with delivery of too much intervention (Saini et al., 2017).

As the broad investments in the biomedical strategy of tackling the threat of cancer have gained sound footing, concerns have been uttered that this transfer in priorities leaves public health approaches underestimated and progressively underfinanced (Bayer and Galea, 2015). Several reports suggests that the biggest potential for global reduction of cancer-related morbidity and mortality might still be retrievable through well-organised and executed strategies for primary prevention of cancer, as up to 50% of premature onset of cancer cases and premature cancer deaths are attributed to preventable causes (GBD 2015 Risk Factors Collaborators, 2016; Schottenfeld et al., 2013; Vineis and Wild, 2014). We know that the progress we have witnessed in life quality and life expectancy throughout the last century is complex and composite, and a result of comprehensive and pervasive changes in how we organized our society. It is in part related to the general increase in human prosperity, facilitating improved public and private infrastructure and education, that were collectively responsible for securing safety and security for most humans by the end of the century (Preston, 1975). Further we know that tobacco and obesity are two of the strongest risk factors for premature death, both caused by cardiovascular disease and cancer. We know that the use of tobacco and unhealthy dietary habits are strongly correlated to socioeconomic discrepancies, where income, education and living conditions are strong predictive factors, even in high- and very-high-income countries (McCartney et al., 2013). Globally there remains a vast unreleased potential for health benefits by public health strategies. Promoting equality and emergence from poverty, we can potentially enforce the recourses needed for individuals to make health-promoting lifestyle choices throughout their lives, reducing the risk for premature morbidity and mortality, not only from cancer but also from other causes. However, one should be aware that implementation of encompassing biomarker strategies, precision oncology or ultimately personalised medicine might also contribute to increased inequality, at least on the global scale.

4. Introspection as an instrument for obtaining a meaningful goal of victory

Focusing on the development and evolvement of the cancer biomarker field through the last 45 years we can look back at several battles overcome and rejoice in multiple victories representing pivotal milestones in our biological understanding of the world we live in. Implementation and adaptation of cancer biomarkers, precision oncology and the anticipation of personalised medicine have further contributed in the evolution of expectations, values, healthcare services, priorities and politics. Simultaneously we may sense that all of the implications caused by the expansion of this discipline were not initially foreseen, intended or even considered desirable. Summarizing some of the collateral and unintentional effects caused by 45 years of warfare, we can identify indications of enforced reductionism and bio-medicalisation within the practice of medicine. This shift is gradually shaping our approach for preventing, diagnosing, and treating disease. Eventually it might even contribute to tendencies of developing and delivering more healthcare services than demonstrated beneficial (Brownlee et al., 2017), possibly at the cost of other favourable strategies. Such harmful effects are difficult to assess, but we should be attentive to the possibility that they might contribute to a general culture of bio-socialisation and an almost boundless expansion of medicine in our societies, resulting in the introduction of novel hazards, harms and forms of suffering (Clarke et al., 2003). We are all potential losers of this process; the general public, our local cultures and our societies. If we are not attentive there may ultimately be only losers in this war.

In military warfare there are international directives aiming at protecting both combatants and civilians, with the overall objective of alleviating the adversities of war, reducing unwarranted suffering and destruction. Maybe we should discuss whether such considerations should be contemplated also in the 'war on cancer', and the expansion of the cancer biomarker field to limit unintentional damage. Our primary challenge is that we have no clear endpoints in our war. It is unclear when to be satisfied with our achievements, or what it takes for us to admit that the cause is lost. If we want to retain the idea that we can successfully cure all cancers or relieve all its associated suffering, we should probably be prepared for a very long withstanding conflict.

In the 6th century BC the famous Chinese general Sun Tzu wrote in his book 'The Art of War': "If you know the enemy and know yourself, you need not fear the result of a hundred battles. If you know yourself but not the enemy, for every victory gained you will also suffer a defeat. If you know neither the enemy nor yourself, you will succumb in every battle" (Tzu, 5th century BC). We have spent the last 45 years gradually getting to know our enemy, cancer. We have come a long way in untangling its identity and impact on human society and human biology. One might however argue that throughout this process we have endangered vital knowledge about our true selves. Application of biomedical methods presupposes that we fragment the subject we are attempting to clarify, maybe compromising our ability to illuminate the matter evenly and simultaneously from all angles. Gradually this trade-off might have contributed to the loss of overview of our own forces and motives, and it might additionally have facilitated an endorsement of reductionism and medicalisation, propensities that ultimately might threaten human health and wellbeing. Perhaps Sun Tzu made a point we should take into account if we want to have the possibility to win the 'war on cancer' in a way that is meaningful and empowering, serving a true health benefit for humanity. The vital step in retrieving our balance may therefore be to take a step back and take a good and thorough view in the mirror, where the scope of the introspection is to shed light on why we as a community and single individuals think that cancer represents such a threat that a war is warranted at all (Hodgkin, 1985; Annas, 1995).

Both cancer incidence and cancer-related mortality rates are inescapably continuously rising. Predictions based on anticipated global demographic changes, like population growth and change in age distribution, indicate that cancer might soon be the biggest "killer" of all human diseases (Thun et al., 2010). This is often the initial declaration about the hazards of cancer, appealing to our coherence and commitment to the 'cancer war'. Despite unsettling results within the cancer field however, we should retain and rejoice in the fact that public health has continuously improved since the 1970s, and life expectancy has steadily increased. We have witnessed an impressive decrease in morbidity and mortality related to infections and cardiovascular diseases worldwide, constituting a grand shift towards increased cancer specific mortality. The demographic change, triggered by the same progress, is consequently one of the foremost momentums causing a rise in cancer incidence. Cancer is mainly a disease of the elderly, and as our populations age the occurrence of cancer surges (GBD 2013 Mortality and Causes of Death Collaborators, 2015; Stewart and Wild, 2014). The rise is additionally supported by the development and implementation of extensive diagnostic strategies, assuring that no cancer-specific health impairment or cancer-specific death remains obscure. We have implemented systematic screening programs and established tests that are utilised in unsystematic screening for cancer. Incidental findings of solid or liquid tumours, associated with examination for other, unrelated medical conditions, further add to the frequency (Welch and Black, 2009). Although an increase in cancer incidence and cancer-related mortality is factual and poses a serious challenge to healthcare delivery organisations and welfare systems across the globe, paradoxically the extent of the challenge posed by cancer largely reflects both human and technological progress.

Concurrently it is important to remember that despite this progress we remain mortal in absolute terms, independently of shifts in causes of mortality. This sobering element may unconditionally limit the benefit rewarded by preventing or curing all cancer. If we are fighting a war on cancer because we do not want to die from cancer, but rather from something else, we must be frank and ask ourselves why this is so.

Although we have not managed to cure advanced cancer, we have made huge improvements concerning care and symptom relief in cancer patients. Death by cancer is therefore not unavoidably associated with graver suffering than death by other diseases, like heart failure, obstructive lung disease or degenerative neurological diseases. Despite a myriad of other serious and devastating human conditions, there are however few that evoke such an emotional response as cancer. Is it so that cancer holds a special position among human diseases in a socio-cultural context? And if so, how and why did it happen?

Although the military rhetoric applied throughout this chapter is meant only as a metaphor, it describes the approach to the challenge of cancer and captures how many talk and communicate about cancer, both in the clinic, within cancer research communities, in politics and in the mainstream media (Skott, 2002; Vrinten et al., 2014). As our way of understanding the world depends on concepts and metaphors, the rhetoric style we have adopted talking about cancer might have contributed in the creation of an image of cancer as a malicious and erratic enemy that should be dreaded and feared. We should therefore reflect on our phrasing of words as the language we use actually might promote increased fear of cancer and a feeling of defeat when faced with death. If we are more scared of cancer than other diseases, this might be part of the suffering related to the condition, adding to the physical challenges in itself (Clarke and Everest, 2006, Malm, 2016; Penson et al., 2004).

Maybe the 'war on cancer' is ultimately only a small piece in a more obscure and unarticulated confrontation with fear itself, triggered by uncertainty and our own mortality (Heath, 2014). Perhaps the fear is additionally reinforced and sustained by hope and the promise of increased control (and maybe even immorality?) in the near future, promoted and disseminated by techno-scientific solutions and medical advancements? While risk reduction seems to be our primary combat strategy, the realistic outcome of such a war might unavoidably be total and raw defeat. Although risk reduction is a powerful weapon, there are limits to its range, and consequently as medicine has developed as one of our main contemporary tools facilitating risk reduction, there may be boundaries for what power medicine should exert on our lives before it becomes inexpedient. No matter how good we are at predicting and preventing the onset of cancer or any other disease for that matter, or however successful we are at treating it, life is a frail project, and we will ultimately be caught up with by old age, health impairment and death. Possibly there may not be any arms imaginable that could facilitate even a partial victory in this war. Therefore if our true reason and motive for engaging in the conflict is to attempt to improve human life reliably we may have to consider taking some corrective measures.

In the end fear seems like a frail reason for fighting a war. Tackling fear by attempting to 'kill' inflated monsters does not cure terror at its root. If fear of uncertainty and death is a core driver in the 'war on cancer' it might therefore be worth an attempt to reduce the suffering related to cancer by confronting fear at its core, restoring faith in our own ability to cope with adversity and uncertainty. Maybe the standing WHO definition of health, "… a state of complete physical, mental and social well-being and not merely the absence of disease or infirmity" (Constitution of the World Health Organization, 1946), is essentially part of the challenge. Increased biomedical understanding demonstrates that not all pathological processes necessarily couple with a subjective experience of health impairment. "Changing the emphasis towards the ability to adapt and self manage in the face of social, physical, and emotional challenges", a suggestion put forward by Huber and colleagues in 2011 (Huber et al., 2011), offers an attempt of reframing the concept of health in a way that might serve as a more constructive definition for our healthcare research and healthcare services to centre around. This understanding of health ascertains the fact that human life is a process, and that even pain and suffering can add a certain valuable quality to life that might accommodate health in a broader sense. Life altering experiences like facing your own mortality can potentially enforce a potential for growth and meaning (Moreno and Stanton, 2013). Maybe we should not be afraid of acknowledging the value of struggling. Losing parts of oneself is existential. It should hurt and we should probably expect it to hurt. Maybe what we need is the strength to meet our patients and our loved ones and recognize that a situation is bursting with pain, and say that it is okay.

Currently the boundaries of our society are changing faster than most of us can keep track of. Big data, automation, artificial intelligence, synthetic biology, and genetic engineering are just some of the emerging technologies that expand the limits of what we have previously thought possible far beyond imagination. The cancer biomarker field is ultimately just one of these currents, eventually adding up to a powerful and ruthless stream. It is together that these flows eventually form their transformative power on perspectives of health and contemporary identities.

Techno-scientific progress clearly advances the possibilities for predicting, preventing, diagnosing and treating disease. It is however possible that the benefits provided by this development is limited by that fact that we remain vulnerable and mortal. In the excitement of the prospects the future might offer us, let us not forget what is at stake: our perception of concepts like health and disease, wellness and suffering, life and death. These are all concepts that shape our personal and collective identities, and our interactions. The challenge of finding the balance point between over-treatment and therapeutic nihilism is a difficult exercise dating back to Hippocrates himself. The equity between risk reduction as a beneficial and empowering approach versus risk reduction as a diminishing and destructive force remains elusive, although imperative. It is however a focus point we should probably always strive to centre our healthcare services around, minimising iatrogenic effects of individual, social and cultural character. As King Midas believed gold would make his world shine with happiness, let us not reason that a cancer free world would necessarily be a happy world. A world void of pathological processes may equal a disease-free world, but it may not make human life more beautiful.

5. References

Annas, G. J. (1995). Reframing the debate on health care reform by replacing our metaphors. *The New England Journal of Medicine, 332*(11), 744-747.

Bayer, R. and Galea, S. (2015). Public Health in the Precision-Medicine Era. *The New England Journal of Medicine, 373*(6), 499-501.

Breitbart, W. S. and Alici, Y. (2009). Psycho-oncology. *Harvard Review of Psychiatry, 17*(6), 361-376.

Brodersen, J., Schwartz, L. M. and Woloshin, S. (2014). Overdiagnosis: How cancer screening can turn indolent pathology into illness. *Apmis, 122*(8), 683-689.

Brownlee, S., Chalkidou, K., Doust, J., Elshaug, A. G., Glasziou, P., Heath, I., Nagpal, S., Saini, V., Srivastava, D., Chalmers K. and Korenstein D. (2017). Evidence for overuse of medical services around the world. *Lancet*, DOI: 10.1016/S0140-6736(16), 32585-5.

Clarke, A. E., Shim, J. K., Mamo, L., Fosket J. R. and Fishman J. R. (2003). Biomedicalization: Technoscientific transformations of health, illness, and US biomedicine. *American Sociological Review, 68*(2), 161-194.

Clarke, J. N. and Everest, M. M. (2006). Cancer in the mass print media: fear, uncertainty and the medical model. *Social Science & Medicine, 62*(10), 2591-2600.

Chatterjee, S. K. and Zetter, B. R. (2005). Cancer biomarkers: knowing the present and predicting the future. *Future Oncology Journal, 1*(1), 37-50.

Collins, D. C., Sundar, R., Lim J. S. and Yap T. A. (2017). Towards Precision Medicine in the Clinic: From Biomarker Discovery to Novel Therapeutics. *Trends in Pharmacological Sciences, 38*(1), 25-40.

Collins, F. S. and Varmus, H. (2015). A new initiative on precision medicine. *The New England Journal of Medicine, 372*(9), 793-795.

Constitution of the World Health Organization (1946). *American Journal of Public Health and the Nation's Health 36*(11), 1315-1323.

Cyranoski, D. (2016). China embraces precision medicine on a massive scale. *Nature, 529*(7584), 9-10.

Druker, B. J., Talpaz, M., Resta, D. J., Peng, B., Buchdunger, E., Ford, J. M., Lydon, N. B., Kantarjian, H., Capdeville, R., Ohno-Jones, S. and Sawyers C. L. (2001). Efficacy and safety of a specific inhibitor of the BCR-ABL tyrosine kinase in chronic myeloid leukemia. *The New England Journal of Medicine, 344*(14), 1031-1037.

Elenko, E., Underwood L. and Zohar D. (2015). Defining digital medicine. *Nature Biotechnology, 33*(5), 456-461.

GBD 2013 Mortality and Causes of Death Collaborators (2015). Global, regional, and national age-sex specific all-cause and cause-specific mortality for 240 causes of death, 1990-2013: a systematic analysis for the Global Burden of Disease Study 2013. *Lancet, 385*(9963), 117-171.

GBD 2015 Risk Factors Collaborators (2016). Global, regional, and national comparative risk assessment of 79 behavioural, environmental and occupational, and metabolic risks or clusters of risks, 1990-2015: a systematic analysis for the Global Burden of Disease Study 2015. *Lancet*, *388*(10053), 1659-1724.

Global Alliance for Genomics and Health (2016). A federated ecosystem for sharing genomic, clinical data. *Science*, *352*(6291), 1278-1280.

Gøtzsche, P. C. and Jorgensen, K. J. (2013). Screening for breast cancer with mammography. *The Cochrane Database of Systematic Reviews*, *6*, DOI: 10.1002/14651858.CD001877.pub5.

Hanahan, D. (2014). Rethinking the war on cancer. *Lancet*, *383*(9916), 558-563.

Hanahan, D. and Weinberg, R. A. (2000). The hallmarks of cancer. *Cell*, *100*(1), 57-70.

Hanahan, D. and Weinberg, R. A. (2011). Hallmarks of cancer: the next generation. *Cell*, *144*(5), 646-674.

Heath, I. (2014). Role of fear in overdiagnosis and overtreatment--an essay by Iona Heath. *British Medical Journal*, *349*, DOI: 10.1136/bmj.g6123

Hodgkin, P. (1985). Medicine is war: and other medical metaphors. *British Medical Journal (Clinical Research Edition)*, *291*(6511), 1820-1821.

Huber, M., Knottnerus, J. A., Green, L., van der Horst, H., Jadad, A. R., Kromhout, D., Leonard, B., Lorig, K., Loureiro, M. I., van der Meer, J. W. M., Schnabel, P., Smith, R., van Weel, C. and Smid, H. (2011). How should we define health? *British Medical Journal*, *343*, DOI: 10.1136/bmj.d4163

Hunter, D. J. (2016). Uncertainty in the Era of Precision Medicine. *The New England Journal of Medicine*, *375*(8), 711-713.

Ilic, D., Neuberger, M. M., Djulbegovic, M. and Dahm, P. (2013). Screening for prostate cancer. *The Cochrane Database of Systematic Reviews*, *1*, DOI: 10.1002/14651858.CD004720.pub3

Institute for Systems Biology (2017). What is systems biology. Retrieved 20th March 2017, from https://www.systemsbiology.org/about/what-is-systems-biology/

Jameson, J. L. and Longo, D. L. (2015). Precision medicine - personalized, problematic, and promising. *The New England Journal of Medicine*, *372*(23), 2229-2234.

McCartney, G., Collins, C. and Mackenzie, M. (2013). What (or who) causes health inequalities: theories, evidence and implications? *Health Policy*, *113*(3), 221-227.

Malm, H. (2016). Military Metaphors and Their Contribution to the Problems of Overdiagnosis and Overtreatment in the "War" Against Cancer. *American Journal of Bioethics*, *16*(10), 19-21.

Mandelli, F., Diverio, D., Avvisati, G., Luciano, A., Barbui, T., Bernasconi, C., Broccia, G., Cerri, R., Falda, M., Fioritoni, G., Leoni, F., Liso, V., Petti, M. C., Rodeghiero, F., Saglio, G., Vegna, M. L., Visani, G., Jehn, U., Willemze, R., Muus, P., Pelicci, P. G., Biondi, A. and Lo Coco, F. (1997). Molecular remission in PML/RAR alpha-positive acute promyelocytic leukemia by combined all-trans retinoic acid and idarubicin (AIDA) therapy. Gruppo Italiano-Malattie Ematologiche Maligne dell'Adulto and Associazione Italiana di Ematologia ed Oncologia Pediatrica Cooperative Groups. *Blood*, *90*(3), 1014-1021.

Marx, V. (2015). The DNA of a nation. *Nature*, *524*(7566), 503-505.

McGranahan, N. and Swanton, C. (2017). Clonal Heterogeneity and Tumor Evolution: Past, Present, and the Future. *Cell*, *168*(4), 613-628.

Meader, N., King, K., Wright, K., Graham, H. M., Petticrew, M., Power, C., White, M. and Sowden, A. J. (2017). Multiple Risk Behavior Interventions: Meta-analyses of RCTs. *American Journal of Preventive Medicine*, DOI: 10.1016/j.amepre.2017.01.032

Mirnezami, R., Nicholson, J.and Darzi A. (2012). Preparing for precision medicine. *The New England Journal of Medicine*, *366*(6), 489-491.

Moreno, P. I. and Stanton, A. L. (2013). Personal growth during the experience of advanced cancer: a systematic review. *The Cancer Journal*, *19*(5), 421-430.

Patterson, J. T. (1988). A Dread Disease: Cancer in Modern American Culture. *The Missouri*

Review, 11(3), 168-178.

Penson, R. T., Schapira, L., Daniels, K. J., Chabner, B. A., Lynch Jr, T. J (2004). Cancer as Metaphor. *The Oncologist, 9*(6), 708-716.

Prasad, V., Fojo, T. and Brada, M. (2016). Precision oncology: origins, optimism, and potential. *Lancet Oncology, 17*(2), e81-86.

Preston, S. H. (1975). The changing relation between mortality and level of economic development. *Population Studies, 29*(2), 231-248.

Roser, M. (2016). Life Expectancy. Retrieved 17th March 2017, from https://ourworldindata.org/life-expectancy/

Saini, V., Garcia-Armesto, S., Klemperer, D., Paris, V., Elshaug, A. G., Brownlee, S., Ioannidis, J. P. and Fisher, E. S. (2017). Drivers of poor medical care. *Lancet*. DOI: 10.1016/S0140-6736(16)30947-3

Schottenfeld, D., Beebe-Dimmer, J. L., Buffler, P. A. and Omenn, G. S. (2013). Current perspective on the global and United States cancer burden attributable to lifestyle and environmental risk factors. *Annual Review of Public Health, 34*, 97-117.

Skott, C. (2002). Expressive metaphors in cancer narratives. *Cancer Nursing, 25*(3), 230-235.

Slamon, D. J., Leyland-Jones, B., Shak, S., Fuchs, H., Paton, V., Bajamonde, A., Fleming, T., Eiermann, W., Wolter, J., Pegram, M., Baselga, J. and Norton, L. (2001). Use of chemotherapy plus a monoclonal antibody against HER2 for metastatic breast cancer that overexpresses HER2. *The New England Journal of Medicine, 344*(11), 783-792.

Stewart B. W., Wild C. P. (2014). *World Cancer Report 2014*. Lyon, France: International Agency for Research on Cancer, World Health Organization.

Tannock, I. F. and Hickman, J. A. (2016). Limits to Personalized Cancer Medicine. *The New England Journal of Medicine, 375*(13), 1289-1294.

Thun, M. J., DeLancey, J. O., Center, M. M., Jemal, A. and Ward E. M. (2010). The global burden of cancer: priorities for prevention. *Carcinogenesis, 31*(1), 100-110.

Vineis, P. and Wild, C. P. (2014). Global cancer patterns: causes and prevention. *Lancet, 383*(9916), 549-557.

Tzu, S. (5th century BC). *The Art of War*. Translated by Lionel Giles in 1910. The Project Gutenberg eBook, Retrieved 10 April 2017, from http://www.gutenberg.org/ebooks/132

Vogt, H., Hofmann, B. and Getz, L. (2016). The new holism: P4 systems medicine and the medicalization of health and life itself. *Medicine, Health Care and Philosophy, 19*(2), 307-323.

Vrinten, C., McGregor, L. M., Heinrich, M., von Wagner, C., Waller, J., Wardle, J. and Black, G. B. (2014). What do people fear about cancer? A systematic review and meta-synthesis. *Lancet, 384*(S12) DOI: http://dx.doi.org/10.1016/S0140-6736(14)62138-3

Wagner, P. D. and Srivastava, S. (2012). New paradigms in translational science research in cancer biomarkers. *Translational Research, 159*(4), 343-353.

Weinstein, I. B. (2002). Cancer. Addiction to oncogenes--the Achilles heal of cancer. *Science, 297*(5578), 63-64.

Welch, H. G. and Black, W. C. (2010). Overdiagnosis in cancer. *Journal of the National Cancer Institute, 102*(9), 605-613.

Weston, A. D. and Hood, L. (2004). Systems biology, proteomics, and the future of health care: toward predictive, preventative, and personalized medicine. *Journal of Proteome Research, 3*(2), 179-196.

8

EXPENSIVE CANCER DRUGS AS A POST-NORMAL PROBLEM

Roger Strand

1. The Issue: Cancer Drugs are Becoming "Too Expensive" for National Health

Several new cancer treatments share the following characteristics: (1) They offer a therapeutic advantage that from a statistical point of view may be more or less marginal, but at the same time may radically improve the length and quality of *some* cancer patients. This yields a promise of clinical benefit to patients and their doctors alike, and in this sense there is a *demand* for these treatments. (2) The treatments are expensive, and typically no less expensive than their predecessors. (3) In countries that we might still wish to call welfare states – Norway and the UK, for example – the availability and affordability of these drugs as part of public health services have become a matter of political contestation in public decision-making institutions as well as in news media and the public sphere. The reason for the politicization of the issue is the coincidence between the high cost and the potentially high benefit of these therapies. They are increasingly perceived as necessary but "too expensive" for public health (see Tranvåg and Norheim, this volume, ch. 4, for an extensive discussion).

When discussing the ethics of cancer treatments and cancer biomarkers, a wide panorama of issues could be imagined. One could and should

Anne Blanchard and Roger Strand (Eds.), *Cancer Biomarkers: Ethics, Economics and Society.* Bergen: Megaloceros Press, 2017. ISBN 978-82-91851-04-4 (paperback). https://doi.org/10.24994/2018/b.biomarkers © The Authors / Megaloceros Press.

discuss issues of global justice and equity, noting that cancer patients in wealthy societies benefit from, or in more candid terms, *spend* more medical resources than patients with less prestigious health problems (for instance mental illnesses) and definitely more than most patients in low-income countries. Taking the view that ethics are not only a matter of discussing what constitutes a right action but also the good life, we could also discuss if and when novel treatments indeed contribute to the good life (and not only a long life that satisfies health-related quality of life measures). For instance, in line with Caroline Engen's reflections (this volume, ch. 7) on the certitude of our own mortality, we might discuss if and when medical treatments do little more than adding time, speed and perhaps even turbulence or chaos to the modern individual's race away from ageing and death (Blanchard, 2016). Perhaps the money is not always so well spent after all, even if some QALYs – quality-adjusted life years – indeed are bought.

Still, the main frame of ethics for novel cancer treatment enters only to a small degree into questions of global equity or alienation from death. It has come to take for granted that the treatments are desirable and that issues of distributive justice are the important ones and that they can be meaningfully discussed and resolved mostly at the national level. In this way, public debate, political decision-making and ethical expertise allow themselves to address the possible rights to new immunotherapies without, say, holding them against the rights of Syrian children (apparently also when those children are entering our own Northern countries). This is the frame to which also several of the chapters of this volume contribute – of distributive justice within a European public health service (Cairns, this volume, ch. 3; Tranvåg and Norheim, this volume, ch. 4) or a US health insurance system (Fleck, this volume, ch. 5). Within this frame a number of legitimate questions emerge, including "What is a legitimate monetary cost for a health benefit?", "How should we measure the costs and benefits?" and "How would issues of distributive justice be affected by the introduction of biomarkers into the decision-making?"

My purpose in stating the obvious is not to criticise this framing of the issues. First of all, different framings will always exist in parallel and it would be futile, unwise and perhaps dangerous to try to police every ethics debate into the ultimate debate about what is right and what is good. This is particularly true for the good: People differ on their conceptions of the good life and will accordingly differ on their views of the dangers of medicalisation. Secondly, "ought" implies "can". Although issues of global justice should not be dismissed simply because there are few means or opportunities currently available to resolve them, local, national and contextual problems cannot and should not be put on hold in the meantime. Finally, we should develop a clear understanding of the ways in which issues are framed in a society before we begin to pass judgements on them. In what follows, I shall briefly review how the issue of 'too expensive' cancer treatments has come to be framed in public discourse in my home country, Norway. The chapter continues with an introduction of the theoretical concepts of post-normal science and applies the normal/post-normal distinction to explain the apparent incommensurability between the official institutional discourse on prioritization of expensive cancer treatments with the mainstream mass media discourse portraying and voicing the outcry of individual patients. Finally, I will discuss possibilities for moving forward, towards conditions for a better social dialogue on these issues.

2.   "The Authorities are Killing Me"

In their seminal paper on biopolitics, Brekke and Sirnes (2011) analysed case studies from Norway and the US and showed how biomedical promises together with patients' hope and despair produce new sources of power in society, to the point at which the Norwegian Parliament changed the legislation on medical biotechnology on the basis of a campaign revolving around the (controversial) medical needs of one single child. Their paper criticised the rather optimistic analyses of sociologists such as Nicholas Rose, who has seen the development of modern medicine and above all genetics as a source of individual empowerment, progress and hope. Indeed, Rose suggested the concept of the 'somatic individual', a modern citizen knowledgeable about the opportunities created by biomedicine and empowered to secure his or her own health with the aid of science. In the eyes of Brekke and Sirnes, public campaigns around fatal diseases display not so much hope as despair over the lack of a cure. What emerges in their view, is the figure of 'the hypersomatic individual' who refuses to accept the fatality of his or her disease and turns to the authorities with the demand that laws should be changed and unlimited resources should be made available so that science can produce the cure. In this way, death by fatal disease is something unacceptable: 'Premature' death becomes a metaphysical tragedy and a moral scandal. The implicit assumption behind this view is that the cure is to be had and science is omnipotent, if only allowed to progress freely. In the words of Brekke and Sirnes: "... the hypersomatic individual is like a volatile concentration of untamed biomedical desires" (2011, p. 358).

Brekke and Sirnes described quite unusual cases and could perhaps, in 2011, have been criticised for theorising on the basis of fringe phenomena. Blanchard (2016) argues that the concept of the hypersomatic individual is becoming ever more relevant and describes quite well how mass media in wealthy countries present and discuss the prioritization issues of expensive cancer treatments, in particular with regard to the promises of immunotherapies. Although Norwegian newspapers show a variety of framings in their coverage on expensive cancer treatments (Strand and Nygaard, 2017), one frequent and powerful frame is the interview with the individual patient who suffers from metastatic cancer and who has been "denied" a certain expensive treatment.

Exactly what "denied" means may vary. It may mean that the particular treatment (and most often a drug) is not offered at all as part of the Norwegian public health service because the authorities have deemed it too expensive or concluded that its effect is not well documented. Alternatively, it may be offered conditional to particular diagnostic and prognostic criteria that are not satisfied by the individual patient in question. It also means that the general policy of not offering the treatment actually has been enforced, that is, the responsible clinician has not administered it anyway by finding a loophole or making an exception with or without a particular reason.

We are then told stories of how these unlucky patients either spend private money or are left to die, stories that insinuate that the authorities are responsible for their death and that this indeed amounts to a moral scandal. The scandal, according to these stories, resides in too little public spending on cancer treatments or health care in general; or applying criteria too strictly; or – interestingly – in displaying inhumane attitudes by giving more importance to money than to human lives. There have been periods in recent years when such news can be found in Norwegian newspapers almost weekly, presenting ill and desperate individuals and their families who are fighting to keep the catastrophe at bay. On the other side of the debate, health authorities, health economists and ethicists explain how the resources for public health care are inevitably limited and that money must be allocated to the benefit of the population as a whole, much along the lines of what has been explained elsewhere in this volume. While fatally ill patients and the health authorities are speaking two very different languages, clinicians and politicians can be found on either of the two sides, depending on the case and the context.

3. Cancer Drugs as a Post-Normal Problem

In the late 1980s and early 1990s, the philosophers Silvio Funtowicz and Jerome Ravetz developed the concept of *post-normal science*. Their first studies analysed cases of technological and environmental risks such as industrial accidents and pollution. In these studies, they came to distinguish between three different states of affairs in terms of risk assessment and management (Funtowicz and Ravetz 1985). In some cases, decision stakes and accompanying uncertainties in the knowledge base for decisions were seen as rather low. This is the zone of applied science or 'normal science':

Scientists can provide a knowledge base that other actors accept as legitimate, and elected or non-elected decision-makers can proceed to deal with the balancing of public interests and values. In other cases, the stakes and/or system uncertainties are too high to be resolved by science alone. This is the zone of technical or professional consultancy, where scientific knowledge has to be supplemented with professional experience and skill. A simple example is that of a medical patient whose health problems are too complex to match the published evidence base and even less so medical textbooks. The experienced clinician will outperform the scientist in such contexts if the case matches his or her experience and he or she is also able to discuss with the patient to find out what is in the patient's best interest. There might be an initial phase of confusion and indecision but gradually doctor and patient will reach a conclusion.

What Funtowicz and Ravetz noted, however, is that some controversies over technological and environmental risks fail to be resolved by applied science and professional consultancy. There can be many features of such cases: There may be complex conflicts of interests, in the sense that there are many different stakeholders who not only have their own stakes in the game but who also disagree on the nature of the issue and on who the legitimate stakeholders are. Funtowicz and Ravetz summarise this situation as *values in dispute*. If stakeholders disagree on the nature of the issue, however, they may also disagree on what the relevant knowledge base is and how reliable and valid it is. *Uncertainties are high*. Still, decisions may be urgent but there is no straight-forward way of resolving the issue. Appealing to science might not help much: What one side accepts as valid expertise, may be seen as insufficient, partisan and illegitimate by the other side. Attempts of using experts to resolve the issue may backfire by entrenching the conflict over the definitions of the issue at stake. This is the post-normal zone, and I think most readers will recognise that controversies over nuclear energy, the Green Revolution, GMOs and climate change are, or have been, situated in this zone.

Since the original publications of Funtowicz and Ravetz an extensive literature on post-normal science (PNS) has emerged. PNS scholars are typically not content with diagnosing various environmental and technological problems as post-normal but also try to devise solutions fit for them. The common denominator of these solutions is to acknowledge the presence of knowledge uncertainty and value plurality as a matter of fact. Especially when decisions are urgent, it may be impossible to eliminate uncertainty in time. PNS approaches would then focus on identifying and characterising that uncertainty rather than trying in vain to eliminate it. Next, one would ask what (imperfect) quality of evidence is sufficient to arrive at a decision. Asking for quality of knowledge rather than "truth" (or conclusive evidence), however, has a democratising potential. Quality of evidence, or "good enough" evidence, is a concept that does not make sense without asking "good enough for what purpose? For whom? Who judges the quality? Who are entitled to judge?" What is seen empirically in post-normal cases is that stakeholders and concerned citizens claim to have a say in what arguably is also a political issue, namely the choice of the purpose and the recognition of legitimate stakeholders. According to the PNS literature, they are right in doing so: There is no reason to believe that the decision-making process gets "better" (whatever that means) by closing and insulating it from the scrutiny and participation of civil society.

I believe that the issue of "too expensive" cancer drugs displays several of the features of post-normal problems. Allow me to stereotype and imagine two main sets of actors: On one hand there is the 'establishment', consisting of an elite of non-elected public decision-makers (bureaucrats and appointed experts within the administrative institutions of the public health services) allied with members of government and academic experts especially within medical ethics, health economics and to some extent medical sciences. On the other hand there are the hypersomatic individuals, who are individual persons who construct and present themselves in a certain way to the public sphere in close collaboration with mass media and at times with allied clinicians, patient organisations and perhaps industrial interests. Now, in the conflict between these two sets of actors, values are undoubtedly in dispute and decisions are urgent: The hypersomatic individuals are fatally ill and accuse the establishment of literally killing them. Furthermore, the knowledge base, particularly when it comes to novel treatments, is often incomplete, uncertain and in dispute. The uncertainty may express itself in prioritization committees concluding that the effect (or cost-effectiveness) of a certain treatment is not yet properly documented, while the other side points to published (but perhaps small) clinical trials. The uncertainty is also related to difficult stratification issues. A drug might not be considered cost-effective for a certain diagnosis or a group of patients holding that diagnosis, but a sub-group (or even an individual) may argue that they have good reasons and even evidence (for instance a biomarker) to believe that they will profit much more than the average group from the treatment. And as is often the case in post-normal problems, one can observe that the disagreements are not only between expert and lay; it is also a case of scientific experts opposing each other.

4. Normal Solutions and the Veil of Ignorance

Substantial efforts have been made to renormalise or "modernise" the problem by setting up institutional bodies and procedures for health priority setting in welfare states. Tranvåg and Norheim (this volume, ch. 4) introduces basic principles and practices for priority setting. Although variations and disagreements exist, for instance on how to measure health benefits, how to weigh in the severity of disease, which criteria to deem relevant or irrelevant, et cetera, the underlying principles are mostly consequentialist and definitely always concerned with fairness and reason in the broadest sense. I have never come across variants of ethics or economics for health priority setting that explicitly violated the first key principle mentioned by Tranvåg and Norheim: "Priority setting should be impartial, unprejudiced, and unbiased."

Above, I claimed that such approaches try to 'modernise' the problem. What I mean by that, is that the approach tries to solve the problem in the way that modern societies aim at doing: basing decisions on universal principles founded on reason and rationality that can easily be applied as rules.

It should be noted how well ethics and economics can talk to each other in the context of health priority setting. Usually there is a strong tension between ethics and economics, above all with micro-economics that model human behaviour as self-interested maximisation of own utility. In the field of health priority setting, medical ethicists and health economists understand each other's language and work together for the goal of fair distribution and maximisation of public health. To the extent that welfare states are able to create modern institutions to deal with such issues, it is this language – a logic for fair and rational management of converting capital into health – that is the foundation of the relevant expertise.

From the perspective of this expertise, the hypersomatic individual, crying for unlimited resources for himself or herself, or the clinician crying for his or her patient, or the politician yielding to the media-created pressure, is violating the key principle of priority setting and as such fails to present a valid point of view. The individual patient may not be said to be irrational because he or she might be acting in accordance with own interests, but what he or she says is not relevant for the priority setting process. Indeed, it would be cruel to demand impartiality of a fatally ill patient, and accordingly, individual patients are not relevant participants in priority setting at the general level.

It is relevant to distinguish between general priority setting and individual clinical decisions. Strictly speaking, the destiny of the individual patient is an outcome of the latter and not the former. A patient could be very well helped by a clinician making an exception from the rule, and everybody knows that exceptions are made for a variety of reasons. From the 'modernised' point of view, however, such exceptions are highly problematic. An important part of an ethical framework based on universal principles is that these principles must be followed. Strict rule-following is seen as necessary for fairness and justice. For this reason the two levels of general priority setting and individual clinical decisions are entangled and cannot be isolated from each other.

Tranvåg and Norheim (this volume, ch. 4) describe the framework of accountability for reasonableness, which is somewhat more sophisticated in philosophical terms than what I have described above and might be able to account better for the perspective of the actual patient. Still, I think it is relevant to reflect upon what is assumed by the demand that priority setting should be impartial, unprejudiced and unbiased. One way of understanding what this could mean, is to think in terms of the philosopher John Rawls' concept of 'the veil of ignorance'. The basic idea is that bias should be abstracted away from discussions about fairness and justice. For instance, if I happen to know that I will develop a certain disease in 10 years, I might be inclined to argue in favour of better health services for that disease, out of purely selfish motives. But that is not fair. So in order to make a fair priority decision, I should either not take part in that decision (because I cannot avoid being partial and biased), or some kind of procedure must be implemented to control for that bias. That procedure would amount to the 'veil of ignorance': Somehow, individually or collectively, we have to look upon the matter at hand through a veil that clouds and brackets off any knowledge of our own personal needs and interests. As a society we could implement the veil of ignorance for instance by mainly involving healthy persons in decisions on health priorities, assuming that they have no interests or stakes in particular diseases. In fact, this is even implemented down to the level of the elaboration of the knowledge base by preferring healthy persons or at least a sample of the general population to "score" health states, that is, evaluate through imagined time trade-offs the quality of life of health states resulting from various diseases and illnesses. Patients suffering from these diseases and illnesses are considered unfit because they are 'biased' in their assessments.

From within this expert language, arguments about bias make perfect sense. Considering the distrust and rage against the authorities that can be observed in the media, however, it is quite clear that from the point of view of the suffering patient and particularly the hypersomatic individual, these arguments make no sense. It seems important to try to understand this rage without necessarily agreeing or passing judgement on it, and I will allow myself to speculate on the issue.

From the perspective of the suffering patient, the arguments about bias effectively imply that those who are most affected by the decisions are excluded from taking part in them. Even worse: It is exactly the fact of being directly and severely affected by the decision that disqualifies them from taking part in it. The situation is not unique – it is reminiscent of the logic of jurisprudence and also of certain areas of distributive justice in public administration where interests are taken as bias (research funding for example). Still, it seems strange and counter-intuitive that whoever holds a strong personal stake should be disqualified from taking part in the decision process that affects him or her so strongly, to the level of life or death.

Accordingly, hypersomatic individuals might perceive the situation as paradoxical: Modern society empowers them to create their own careers, families, households and living conditions and democratically influence the development of their own communities and societies. However, when they arrive at the critical point in their lives – perceived as a life and death decision over a certain immunotherapy – they no longer have a say as citizens at the general level of priority setting because they are affected and therefore not impartial and rational (although they might have a say as patients, negotiating with the responsible clinician). It is not surprising that they (or others) come to think of this as David the cancer patient's fight against the Goliath of the health institutions, or perhaps as the fight of vulnerable and mortal humans against a cold and cynical machine.

5. Possible Post-Normal Solutions

I believe to have shown above that the key principles underlying health priority setting, however rational and reasonable, contribute to a climate of distrust between the establishment and hypersomatic individuals. Sometimes the distrust merely manifests itself in public outcries in the media. Occasionally, it escalates and translates into political power to create some kind of exception from the normal and modern principles and practices. One example is the creation of a cancer drugs fund in the UK National Health Service (Linley and Hughes, 2013). Another is the direct instruction from the Norwegian Minister of Health in 2013, Jonas Gahr Støre, to override the national priority decision body and provide ipilimumab to patients with malignant melanoma (Wyller, 2014). This is biopolitics in action.

I do not intend to pass judgement on the described states of affair. The fact that some disagree with or distrust a public institution does not imply that it should be changed. Likewise, the occasional manifestations of biopolitics into what may appear as illogical or inconsequential political actions are not necessarily signs that something is wrong. Perhaps such eruptions can be seen as safety valves in a complex and inevitably imperfect system. Støre, for instance, would be likely to defend his decision of exception as being based on (alternative) expert advice and not as a result of public pressure. There is nothing unique in having public decision-making processes founded upon normative principles of fairness and justice that are quite rigid and idealised, but practiced with some degree of discretion (Bærøe, 2009) or even messiness (Strand and Cañellas-Boltà, 2006) to prevent it from becoming an iron cage bureaucracy.

At the same time, we should be prepared for a development of ever more hypersomatic individuals appealing to the media and the public for the exception that will save their lives. One could imagine a scenario in which the accountability and fairness of the public health system, perhaps the most important value of the entire welfare state, is lost to a type of heated power politics in which access to expensive treatments becomes a matter of the largest and wildest public outcry in news and social media. To use a metaphor from first aid training: On the accident scene, the quietest person is likely to be in the gravest situation. Those who can scream, are stronger, and in the media their voice may be amplified with the resources of other and less obvious interests (such as pharmaceutical industry).

Post-normal approaches typically try to find a third way, defending the role of dialogue and reason without taking for granted that the Establishment should have a monopoly to demarcate between reason and passion and between facts and values. Public outcries against the institutions of the Establishment are not necessarily wrong or unreasonable. I think there could be two types of post-normal approaches to the issue being discussed here: those of knowledge assessment and those of reframing the issue.

As explained above, post-normal knowledge assessment methodologies and approaches take as their point of departure the questions about quality of knowledge – quality for what, for whom, judged by whom and by which criteria? – and they will always consider to extend the peer community by including stakeholders, affected parties and other non-scientists in their capacity as knowledge bearers. To be a bit simplistic, post-normal knowledge assessment takes almost the opposite attitude of 'evidence-based medicine', at least in the most rigid variants of the latter, clinging to some predefined evidence hierarchy. At least since the beginning of the HIV/AIDS epidemic there have been patient-activist groups that have had a strong will to contribute to the knowledge production that ultimately might save their lives, not only by being passive donors of data and biological material but as active co-researchers with their own views on e.g. study design. The point of mentioning the history of HIV/AIDS is not to argue that transdisciplinary dialogue or research, bringing together "normal" scientists with an extended peer community, is a certain path to success. The point is simply that the primary interest of academic, normal science is to accumulate knowledge and above all do so by avoiding falsities to be blended into the knowledge base, for instance by being cautious about claiming positive correlations or causal relationships in the absence of statistically convincing evidence. (For ongoing discussions about the successes and failures of science to do so, see: Ioannidis, 2016.) The difference between academic interests and applied contexts and interests may for instance translate into differences on the trade-off between statistical Type 1 and Type 2 errors and in general on methodological questions about specificity, sensitivity and design. Biomarkers are not irrelevant in this context. When a particular treatment is rendered "too expensive" (in the sense of cost per QALY) for a particular indication, this will mean that the cost-effectiveness is too poor on average for a defined group of patients (for instance those who have a certain diagnosis, or a diagnosis and some other traits including biomarkers). We may imagine an interesting strategy for the group of hypersomatic individuals, if we can think of them as a group, where they argue less for increased over-all costs or more scientific research in general, and rather advocate for more biomarker research so that one could stratify the indications to a greater extent and thereby increase the average cost-effectiveness for some groups. These groups would be smaller, then, so one could also imagine that some subgroups would "lose" by this strategy, if it can be called a loss to not be given a treatment that is unlikely to have a positive effect. The overall vision, however, is not so different from the imaginary of personalised medicine explained by Blasimme (this contribution, ch. 6). It is a future where patients become somewhat empowered by being more involved in the knowledge production and perhaps also influencing it in their own best interest. Indeed, there are already examples of networking and crowd-sourcing of health information among cancer patients and survivors but so far it is difficult to see that they differ from normal science in their methods and outcomes.

Even if the knowledge production becomes post-normal, I think this is not enough to 'solve' the issue of the tension between the Establishment's goal of cost-effectiveness in public health and the desperation of hypersomatic individuals. We may improve the game of public health resource allocation by removing some imperfections but it remains a zero sum game unless society allows the cost per capita to continue to increase. In effect, we are still within a framing of the issue that is experienced as tragic by a number of individuals that is likely to increase with the development of ever more expensive treatments.

Is it at all thinkable to reframe the issue? Could we ask: In which framings does the issue cease to be tragic? I can think of some alternative framings. The two first ones seem less promising but I will mention them anyway.

First, as a matter of fact it is possible to think of the total budget for public health as without limits. In Norway, there have been high-ranking politicians up until recent years who boldly claimed that nobody ought to die in our country because of budget limitations in public health. The claim is totally unrealistic, of course, if taken as absolute. However, the individual patient or clinician does not have to take it as that. They could rightly argue that what they need is just a small extra increase. This does not solve the issue in general and in principle, but it might do it for that individual; I suspect this also happens by clinicians simply using their own judgement and providing a treatment that is beyond what is normally provided, perhaps making up some kind of justification that they might or might not believe themselves. In a way, this is care ethics at work, the doctor crossing boundaries to help his or her patient (or indeed the system allowing pockets of clinicians' discretion). It amounts to care and mercy and, from the patient perspective, luck, at the expense of fairness and justice. The limits to growth in the health budgets (or alternatively, the deficit in the resulting accounts) are not known; ultimately this is a political question.

Secondly, one could imagine the drastic reframing that the certitude of death is abolished and that hypersomatic individuals could rest assured that they are not going to die. This may sound as a joke but as probably all readers of this text know, there is not only a desire for the "Singularity" in certain subcultures but also extensive scientific research taking place that aims at extreme or even indefinite longevity of human life. Optimists who do not think so far might hope for a future where perhaps human longevity is not infinite (an idea so bizarre that it takes another essay to pick it apart and discuss its ecological, social and existential implications) but long enough to abolish 'premature' death. It seems reasonable, however, to expect that the notion of premature death would change as the Bell curve of life expectancies moves towards the right.

Thirdly, one could imagine a reversal of the medicalisation of our culture. There is no reason to think that previous generations have suffered less under disease and death; in a very concrete sense they suffered more as they did not have access to our medical technologies. I take the risk of claiming, however, that the hypersomatic individual and the sense of tragedy of disease and premature death are phenomena that have been constructed relatively recently and that therefore also may be de- and reconstructed. If not by ideology one could imagine by experience: Our civilisation might conclude in the course of a few generations that a thorough medicalisation of our existence coupled with inflated fear of death all in all does not provide a good life. If such a learning process is possible – as a kind of reflexive modernisation – I would expect that things have to become more extreme for that learning to take place: As a society, we would have to experience that the negative side effects of medicalisation and fear of death outweigh the benefits. Again, biomarkers are clearly relevant, helping us to understand when a treatment is expected to be worth it, in terms of the good life, and when it is not.

Last, but definitely not least, one can imagine that the hitherto expensive treatments cease to be so expensive as to challenge health budgets. The prices of many other technologies have indeed decreased drastically over past decades or centuries. What maintains the price level of cancer drugs is the political economy in which the pharmaceutical industry is allowed to earn great profits and taken it at its word when it claims to have large development costs. For those who disbelieve big pharma, the assumption that the drugs have to be expensive is the elephant in the room.

States with political courage could actually change this state of affairs. They could nationalise the industries, diminish or even abolish intellectual property rights, on a large-scale fund public R&D of new cancer treatments, et cetera. In this fourth reframing there is clearly a promising place for biomarkers in the narrative, also during the difficult transformation from a global capitalist and exploitative pharmaceutical industry. Today the high price level can only be maintained if the industry is able to offer new and better drugs or other patentable products before the expiry of their currently patented drugs. Medical improvement by new combinations of old and therefore cheap drugs with new and unpatented biomarkers – perhaps even tailor-made to patients' actual needs and concerns through citizen participation in the research – has a potential to change the political economy of the sector and contribute to the reframing and possible resolution of the issue. The reframing is not without its own uncertainties, however. The scientific uncertainty resides in the unknown potential of combinations. Perhaps they will not deliver results in the same way as novel drugs. The more immediate uncertainty, however, is what might happen if brave politicians make decisions that pharmaceutical industry undoubtedly will perceive as a declaration of war.

6. The Potential Role(s) of Biomarkers

In the first chapter of this book, Anne Blanchard and Elisabeth Wik asked the seemingly simple question "What is a good biomarker?" and arrived at the conclusion that a biomarker should be "good enough":

So the questions we should keep in mind are: for my purpose, what is a 'good enough' biomarker? [...] This is the role of 'good enough' biomarkers: to help reintroduce some human judgement – 'realism', 'reason', 'sensibility' and 'prudence' – (Callahan, 2003) into discussions of what we want from cancer research and care, when faced with our own certain mortality, and rich biological and social complexities.

The post-normal approach is to ask "good enough for what purpose?" Above, I have tried to identify some possible purposes, taking as my point of departure the ethical and social issue at stake rather than the biology of cancer.

What makes a biomarker useful for a post-normal knowledge assessment approach to the tension between the Establishment and the hypersomatic individuals who perceive the authorities to be killing them? How may a biomarker help if we try to reframe the issue, finding a frame that avoids the sense of tragedy without producing a lot of other negative side effects?

For the first purpose – the knowledge assessment – the concept of a good biomarker would be quite close to the normal scientific one. A good biomarker would help stratifying more and better, reducing the standard deviation of the effect of the treatment within the different patient subgroups. The effect could be thought of as clinical benefit but not only that: quality of the remainder of life in the widest sense would be relevant, and perhaps more quality as defined by patients rather than the standard assessments (time trade-offs et cetera by non-patients). One could imagine interesting research projects combining biomarkers, treatments and qualitative studies of living with terminal cancer, including what is important to be able to do during the last phase and how much time it requires.

Perhaps it is also possible to think of a development of packages of biomarkers and tailored treatments with the ambition to counter-act the inflated fear of death. Again, qualitative studies, understanding of terminal cancer, would be called for. Knowing average time spans until progression is important but not sufficient. If we accept the certitude of death, the problem with cancer is not death but suffering and fear of suffering. It is entirely possible to imagine that inter- and transdisciplinary research could develop medical knowledge that integrated biomarkers and treatments with broader knowledge for understanding the psychosomatic, social and existential dimensions of cancer. Indeed, this type of broad knowledge is already there in the form of the personal, unsystematic experience of oncologists who deal on a daily basis with terminal patients who are very much in doubt whether to subject themselves to yet another round of chemotherapy. The question "Is it worth it?" is of course an existential one, but one could dream of biomarkers that substantially simplified the challenge of answering it and helped patients to fight the worthwhile fights and avoid the quixotic ones.

Finally, and no less important, biomarkers could play a key role in challenging the global capitalist and exploitative political economy of cancer drugs. To do that, biomedical research needs to explore more intensively the prospects of combining inexpensive biomarkers with known drugs with expired or expiring patents. In my limited personal experience, the scientists are more than ready; the main challenge belongs to governmental authorities who would need to build the courage to provide sufficient public funding for public knowledge and resist the pressure from capitalist actors who surely will oppose.

7. References

Blanchard, A. (2016). Mapping ethical and social aspects of cancer biomarkers. *New Biotechnology, 33*(6), 763-772.

Brekke, O. A. and Sirnes, T. (2011). Biosociality, biocitizenship and the new regime of hope and despair: interpreting "Portraits of Hope" and the "Mehmet Case". *New Genetics and Society, 30*(4), 347-374.

Bærøe, K. (2009). *Delegated discretion: A call for reasonableness in surrogate decision-making and clinical judgment.* Doctoral dissertation. Bergen, Norway: University of Bergen.

Funtowicz, S. and Ravetz, J. (1985) Three types of risk assessment: a methodological analysis. In Whipple, C. and Covello, V. T. (Eds.), *Risk Analysis in the Private Sector* (pp. 217-231). New York and London: Plenum Press.

Ioannidis, J. P. A. (2016) Why Most Clinical Research Is Not Useful. *PLoS Medicine, 13*(6), e1002049.

Linley, W. G. and Hughes, D. A. (2013) Societal views on NICE, Cancer Drugs Fund and value-based pricing criteria for prioritising medicines: a cross-sectional survey of 4118 adults in Great Britain. *Health Economics, 22*(8), 948-964.

Strand, R. and Cañellas-Boltà, S. (2006). Reflexivity and Modesty in the Application of Complexity Theory. In A. Guimarães Pereira, S. Vaz and S. Tognetti (Eds.), *Interfaces between Science and Society* (pp. 100-117). Sheffield, UK: Greenleaf Publishing.

Strand, R. and Nygaard, I. H. (2017). Narratives of expensive cancer treatments. A study of Norwegian newspapers 2010-2015. In preparation.

Wyller, T. B. (2014). Politics or quasi-science? *Tidsskrift for Den norske lægeforening [Journal of the Norwegian Medical Association], 134,* 320.

.

ABOUT THE AUTHORS

Anne Blanchard is a post-doctoral researcher in Science and Technology Studies at the Centre for the Study of the Sciences and the Humanities, University of Bergen, Norway. Her initial research focussed on decision-making processes around complex and uncertain environmental issues, such as the mobilisation of interdisciplinary science on climate change (PhD in 2011 titled 'Reflexive Interdisciplinarity'), the facilitation of participatory processes around the contentious 'oil-fish debate' in Lofoten, northern Norway (Norwegian-funded UncAP project), or the co-production of 'post-normal' early monsoon knowledge with communities in northeast Bangladesh (Norwegian-funded TRACKS project).

In 2014, this interest developed into increased attention on how to engage in responsible research and innovation, especially in biomedical research, when Anne Blanchard started her post-doc as part of the Centre for Cancer Biomarkers (CCBIO). She looks at the Ethical, Legal and Social Aspects (ELSA) of cancer biomarkers, and is particularly interested in how the various challenges of oncology research (the complexity of cancer biology, challenges of reproducibility and validation of results) impact the broader social, economic and political spheres (see *Mapping ethical and social aspects of cancer biomarkers* (New Biotechnology, 2016) and *Mouse models: some reflections from the lab* (Wageningen Academic Publishers, 2016)).

Alessandro Blasimme is a researcher at the Health Ethics and Policy Lab of the University of Zurich (Switzerland). His research revolves around ethical and policy issues in regenerative medicine, precision medicine and digital health. In particular, he investigates the mutual constitution of novel medical paradigms, evidentiary standards, regulatory processes and public health policy.

Alessando Blasimme studied Philosophy and Bioethics in Rome (Italy) and received a PhD in Bioethics from the European School of Molecular Medicine (University of Milan – Italy). He also received training in science and technology studies (STS) and molecular cell biology. Before joining the University of Zurich, he held a post-doctoral appointment at Inserm (the

French National Institute of Health and Medical Research) and a Fulbright-Schuman research fellowship at Harvard University (STS Program).

His work has appeared in journals such as BMC Medical Ethics, Perspectives in Biology and Medicine, Studies in History and Philosophy of Science, and the American Journal of Bioethics, and he presented his work at more than 40 national and international conferences. He also served as a consultant to the Swiss Academy of Medical Sciences and to French Parliamentary Office for the Evaluation of Scientific and Technological Decisions (OPECST).

John Cairns is Professor of Health Economics at the London School for Hygiene & Tropical Medicine. He is an Associate PI at the Centre for Cancer Biomarkers at the University of Bergen. He has a particular interest in the use of economic information to inform health care decision-making and has been a member of the NICE Appraisal Committee since 2003 and the Scottish Medicines Consortium (2003-2009). He was the health economist on the advisory committee on Safety of Blood, Tissues and Organs 2008-2017, chair of the Department of Health Cost-Effectiveness Methodology for Immunisation Programmes and Procurements working group (2014-16), and member of the working group Assessing the Value of NIHR investment in Systematic Reviews and in Cochrane activities (2015-16). He has been a member of the Department of Health Appraisal Alignment Working Group (since 2014). His research interests include the economic evaluation of cancer treatments, and methods for eliciting preferences over health states and alternative means of delivering healthcare.

Caroline Engen obtained an M.D. from the University of Bergen in 2013. The same year she commenced on her PhD project at UiB, which she is currently working on under the supervision of Professor Bjørn Tore Gjertsen. Her research project aims to elucidate aspects of clonal heterogeneity and clonal evolution in acute myeloid leukemia, with specific focus on possible therapeutic implications.

Leonard M. Fleck, Ph.D., is currently a Professor of Philosophy and Medical Ethics in the Philosophy Dept. (College of Arts and Letters) and in The Center for Ethics and Humanities in the Life Sciences (College of Human Medicine), Michigan State University. He is now in his thirty-second year at Michigan State. He received his Ph.D. in Philosophy from St. Louis University in 1975.

Leonard Fleck's main areas of teaching and research are medical ethics, health care policy, social and political philosophy. He has published over 120 articles, either as book chapters or in various professional journals of philosophy and medical ethics. His most recent major research project is a book titled *Just Caring: Health Care Rationing and Democratic Deliberation* (Oxford University Press, 2009) (480 pp.). He is co-editor of the volume *Fair Resource Allocation and Rationing at the Bedside* (Oxford University Press, 2014), and he is working on a new book about ethical issues related to cutting-edge genetic technologies with the working title *Precision Medicine/ Ethical Ambiguity: Wicked Problems, Ragged Edges, and Rough Justice.* In 2003 he was honoured with a University Distinguished Faculty Award by Michigan State University as well as a Distinguished Faculty Award from the College of Human Medicine.

Ole Frithjof Norheim is a physician and professor in medical ethics, Department of Global Public Health and Primary Care, University of Bergen, and adjunct Professor at the Department of Global Health and Population, Harvard TH Chan School of Public Health. Norheim's wide-ranging research interests include theories of justice, inequality in health, the ethics of priority setting in health systems and how to achieve Universal Health Coverage as well as the Sustainable Development Goals for health.

He is currently leading the research projects *Priority Setting in Global Health (2012-2016,* funded by NORAD) and *Disease Control Priorities – Ethiopia* (2017-2020, funded by BMGF). He also serves as a member of the *DCP3* Advisory Committee to the Editors.

Norheim has chaired the World Health Organisation's Consultative Group on Equity and Universal Health Coverage (2012-2014), the third Norwegian National Committee on Priority Setting in Health Care (2013-2014), and the 2009 revision of Norwegian Guidelines for Primary Prevention of Cardiovascular Disease.

Norheim has published more than 120 peer-reviewed papers (listed in Medline) in journals such as The Lancet, British Medical Journal, Bulletin of WHO, PlosOne, Health Policy and Planning, Social Science & Medicine, and Journal of Medical Ethics.

Mikyung Kelly Seo is a health economist with more than 10 years of experience in health economics and policy. She holds an MSc in health policy, planning and financing from the London School of Economics (LSE) and the London School of Hygiene, and Tropical Medicine (LSHTM). Her research interest is in assessing the economic value of medical technologies including precision medicine and diagnostics. She has a particular interest in developing a health economic model to assess the cost-effectiveness of cancer biomarkers under development and inform technology developers (or funders) in making decisions for reimbursement or further research investment. Currently, she is a PhD candidate of Health Economics in LSHTM and closely collaborates with the Centre for Cancer

Biomarkers at the University of Bergen. Her research interests include health technology assessment, decision-analytic modelling, value of information analysis, economic evaluations along clinical trials, and evidence synthesis.

Roger Strand originally trained as a natural scientist (with a PhD in biochemistry, 1998), developed research interests in the philosophy of science and issues of scientific uncertainty and complexity. This has gradually led his research into broader areas of social research and philosophy, including questions of policy, decision-making and governance at the science-society interface. Strand is currently Professor at the Centre for the Study of the Sciences and the Humanities at the University of Bergen, Norway and an associate PI at the Centre for Cancer Biomarkers at the University of Bergen. He was a member of the National Research Ethics Committee for Science and Technology in Norway (2006-2013) and Chair of the European Commission Expert Group on Indicators for Responsible Research and Innovation (2014-2015).

Eirik Joakim Tranvåg is a physician and PhD candidate at the Department of Global Public Health and Primary Care, University of Bergen. His PhD project is a collaboration between the Global Health Priorities Research Group and Centre for Cancer Biomarkers, and investigates how biomarkers and patient age influence clinical decisions about new and expensive cancer drugs. His main research interests are priority setting in health, the policy and politics of health care, and measures of health inequality.

Elisabeth Wik is a medical doctor specializing in surgical pathology at the Dept. of Pathology, Haukeland University Hospital. She combines the residency with a postdoc position at Centre for Cancer Biomarkers (CCBIO) at the University of Bergen, Norway. Wik did her PhD on tissue biomarkers in endometrial carcinomas (2013), exploring gene expression microarrays in relation to prognostic markers in this cancer type. This work led her interest into continued work on signature biomarkers, exploring composite biomarkers in omics data. At present, her research is focused on breast cancer, examining tumour microenvironment related gene expression signatures across molecular subtypes of breast cancer. As both a junior scientist and pathologist, aiming for a career where combining science and diagnostic pathology, she promotes the translational bridging between histopathology data and molecular tumour information, aiming to improve cancer diagnostics.

Made in the USA
Columbia, SC
06 August 2018